RAW NUTRITION

Restore Your Health by Eating Raw and Eating Right!

Karyn Mitchell, N.D., Ph.D.

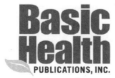

Basic
Health
PUBLICATIONS, INC.

The ideas, recipes, procedures, and suggestions contained in this book are not intended as a substitute for consulting with your physician. We are told that all matters regarding health require medical supervision. Neither the author nor the publisher shall be liable or responsible for any loss, injury, or damage allegedly arising from any information or suggestion in this book. The opinions expressed in this book represent the personal views of the author and you should check with your physician, medical professional, nutritionist, or naturopath before changing your diet. The recipes and information are for educational purposes only and the author assumes no responsibility for any adverse reactions to the information or recipes contained in this book.

Basic Health Publications, Inc.
28812 Top of the World Drive
Laguna Beach, CA 92651
949-715-7327 • www.basichealthpub.com

Library of Congress Cataloging-in-Publication Data.

Mitchell, Karyn.
    Raw nutrition : restore your health by eating raw and eating right! /
Karyn Mitchell.
        p. cm.
    Includes index.
    ISBN 978-1-59120-296-7
    1. Nutrition. 2. Health. 3. Raw food diet. 4. Veganism. 5.
Detoxification (Health) I. Title.
    RA784.M518   2011
    613.2'65—dc23
                                    2011044733

ISBN: 978-1-59120-296-7

Editor: Diana Drew
Typesetting/Book design: Gary A. Rosenberg
Cover design: Mike Stromberg

Printed in the United States of America

10   9   8   7   6   5   4   3   2   1

Contents

To my husband, Steve, my dear sous-chef for over thirty-nine years. Spiritual relationships are essential to life, like the air we breathe. Thank you for sharing this journey of life and for never once asking me, "What is this?"

We're spending $147 billion to treat obesity,
$116 billion to treat diabetes and hundreds of billions
to treat cardiovascular disease and the many types of
cancer that have been linked to the so-called Western diet.
One recent study estimated that 30 percent of the increase
in health-care spending over the past twenty years could
be attributed to the soaring rate of obesity, a condition
that now accounts for nearly a tenth of all spending on
health care. The American way of eating has become the
elephant in the room in the debate over health care.

—MICHAEL POLLAN, *THE OMNIVORE'S DILEMMA*

What You Will Learn in This Book

How food addictions are industry-inspired and emotionally created. How you can heal them by getting your power back and recognizing that stuffed emotions can create weight issues. On a raw vegan diet, most people lose at least ten pounds (4.5 kg) a month eating all they want. It is difficult to remain overweight on a raw-foods diet.

If you are not eating an enzyme-rich, plant-based diet, your body may be stealing enzymes from your pancreas and heart just to digest. This activity of "robbing Peter to pay Paul" can cause diabetes and heart disease. Eating a green salad daily can make a healthy difference in how you look and how you feel every day.

Raw plant enzymes reverse aging. Research and patient studies support this fact.

Are you suffering from malnutrition? Are your children failing to thrive? Are you or your loved ones sick often? Inflammatory processes in the small intestine prevent the absorption of vital nutrients. People who eat only processed foods and fail to eat raw fruits and vegetables may be starving and overeating. More people die in the United States from overeating than undereating.

No one teaches us what we need to eat every day to achieve optimum health and prevent disease. This book gives you an easy-to-remember formula.

Animal foods are not essential forms of vitamins, protein, calcium, amino acids, or essential fats. Most heart-protecting, cancer-fighting, and immune-enhancing substances come from the phytochemicals in plants. Citrus fruits and apples are high in pectin, which helps to lower cholesterol naturally. According to the U.S. Department of Environmental Health:

- Children who ate conventional diets had mean pesticide concentrations in their urine nine times higher than the children who ate organic. Their levels indicated that they had exceeded safe exposure levels set by the Environmental Protection Agency (EPA) and were at increased risk to their health. By contrast, those children who ate organic foods were well within the EPA levels deemed to cause negligible risk.

- Could cancer lose its grip on modern societies if they turned to a balanced vegetarian diet? The answer is yes, according to two major reports, one by the World Cancer Research Fund and the other by the Committee on the Medical Aspects of Food and Nutrition Policy in the United Kingdom.

The McDougall Diet notes: "The truth is that Americans consume six to ten times as much protein as they need. That excess protein overworks the liver and kidneys, causing both these organs to become enlarged and injured. Excess protein consumption causes the kidneys to pull large quantities of calcium from the body, causing bones to weaken and kidney stones to form."

In 1914, an apple contained almost half the daily requirements of iron, but today you would have to eat twenty-six apples to get the same amount of iron. In just under one hundred years, apples have declined in the following: calcium 48 percent, phosphorus 84 percent, iron 96 percent, and magnesium, the heart-helping nutrient, has dropped 82 percent. The amount of calcium in vegetables has also declined: 81 percent in cabbage, 92 percent in lettuce, and 56 percent in spinach. There is little or no iodine or zinc in our produce unless the soils are fed iodine or zinc.

Undiagnosed food allergies create many diseases. Processed foods are the worst offenders. Eating organic, raw vegetables and fruit eliminates many of the antigens that cause allergic reactions and subsequent disease.

Chapter Synopsis

Chapter 1: I have found that many people are afraid to begin a new diet and their concerns range from ensuring their nutritional needs to actually undergoing change. Growing, buying, and storing produce.

Chapter 2: People may look as if they're healthy, based on blood tests, but feel horrible and anxious. I explain how a very simple, raw alkaline diet can help them feel better than they ever imagined. Why organic foods are essential.

Chapter 3: Plant foods provide all that we need in terms of enzymes and nutrition. Vitamin content is given. An explanation of how enzymes are not killed in the stomach only deactivated until later.

Chapter 4: It is not always easy to change old eating habits. Emotional and spiritual ideas to inspire change.

Chapter 5: Research concerning dead, processed foods and their relationship to diseases like cancer. Raw fruits and vegetables contain antioxidants and nutrients that prevent cancer.

Chapter 6: Plant foods contain quality and adequate protein for our daily requirements. A list of protein content of plant-based foods and a comparison to animal protein.

Chapter 7: Learn about conflicts of interest in the food industry: 85 percent of nutrition information taught to school-aged children comes directly from the Dairy Association. Harvard research and the FDA's SAD food pyramid.

Chapter 20: Healing teas and water; teas to drink as remedies for discomfort. Fennel and calendula for intestinal gas.

Chapter 21: Beyond salads: easy recipes to follow and rotate for the three-month healing diet.

Chapter 22: A grocery list of organic foods to purchase on a weekly basis to make preparing raw foods easier.

Chapter 23: Simple and delicious recipes that can change your life.

Chapter 24: Final words of support. If you have a disease, the first consideration for healing is often dietary. Ideas and encouragement for the healing process.

Before a person can be healed, one medicine man told me years after medical school, he or she must answer three simple questions: "Who are you?" "Where did you come from?" and "Why are you here?" This California elder believed that anyone who could give clear answers to these three questions would be well.

—LEWIS MEHL-MADRONA, M.D., *COYOTE MEDICINE*

Tools for Preparing Raw Foods

Many people believe that you need lots of special tools to become a raw chef, and this notion may be intimidating. I suggest that you use the knives, the food processor, graters, the salad spinner, and the blender that you already have. A good health investment comes from making better choices in the produce aisle or farmers' market, not in emptying your pockets to invest in a new kitchen or costly tools. There is one type of tool that you might find beneficial for raw food preparation, but if you do not own this tool, you will still be fine without it. That tool is either a high-powered blender, like a Vita Mix to create healthy smoothies or a juicer. My favorite juicer is a centrifugal type by Breville. Breville's top juicer model allows you to make extra juice that you can store in the refrigerator so you can skip a day or two of juicer cleanup. Enzymes are not destroyed by centrifugal juicers, as they are with the single-gear juicers, so you can store and keep the juice, as opposed to drinking it as soon as possible. This juicer also has a larger tube for feeding fruits and vegetables; a whole apple can be processed at one time. I still suggest that you at least cut apples or pears in half to check for mold. The centrifugal model also is the easiest to clean. Investigate which of these two might be useful for your purposes. With a high-speed blender, you consume all the fiber that is in the vegetable or fruit, and it is truly the quickest of all to clean. A juicer extracts the juice from the pulp and you drink only the liquid, sans fiber. Decide which works best with your particular lifestyle, or forgo the purchase of either and invest your resources in creative raw recipes that abound on the Internet and even in this book. Choose to make this journey a joyous one, but please allow your adult self to be in charge of making healthy food decisions.

Acknowledgments

I would like to acknowledge all the herbalists and naturopaths who have gone before me, and those who will follow, creating and preserving the tradition of botanical medicine. I would like to thank my grandfather, Kenneth Hedlund, who introduced me to herbs as healing allies, and my husband, Steve Mitchell, who, for over two decades, cultivated our acres of medicinal herbs. He tinctured, dried, preserved, and encapsulated organic and hard-to-find botanicals for my patients.

I am grateful to Basic Health Publications, Norman Goldfind, and my most patient and insightful editor, Diana Drew.

Thank you to all of the natural food co-ops and CSAs, especially the three than have been a huge part of our family's health: New Pioneer Co-op (aka "New Pi") in Iowa City and Coralville, which I started to visit at their inception as a student at the University of Iowa; Willie Street Co-op in Madison, Wisconsin; and Duck Soup Co-op in DeKalb, Illinois. Our persistent foraging for fresh organic produce takes us though three Midwestern states. Co-ops are run by diligent, hardworking members who are truly dedicated to health. They understand that what we feed ourselves and what we eat on a daily basis becomes the fertile soil for the seeds for the next generation.

I appreciate and thank Midwest Naturopathic College and the students and interns who are called to pursue not only a profession, but a new way of life in the ancient (not alternative) tradition of naturopathy.

And, last but not least, I am humbly grateful for three generations of patients who entrusted me with their healing process, and then accepted responsibility for their own health.

Introduction

*In this fast-paced world, it is too frequently the case that people
accept what society, family members, and the authorities whom
nobody ever seems to question believe regarding how to live their
lives. And yet, the happiest people I know have been those who
have accepted the primary responsibility for their own spiritual
and physical well-being—those who have inner strength,
courage, determination, common sense, and faith in the process
of creating more balanced and satisfying lives for themselves.*

—ANN WIGMORE, *WHY SUFFER: HOW I OVERCAME ILLNESS
AND PAIN NATURALLY*

Who teaches us what to eat? How do we know that we are eating the
proper nutrients that we need each day to ensure a healthy mind and
body? I was inspired to write this book for those people who have never once
considered what a great diet might look like and yet were afraid to let go of
destructive eating habits. I have heard that the definition of insanity is repeating
the same action time after time and expecting a different outcome. Yet people
expect to get well and stay well while eating the same dead foods every day. I
am writing this book to help you nurture your body with what it most needs to
function well and be disease-free. I want you to be assured that what I am recommending for you is one of humankind's original diets. It is not a fad, nor is it
in any way dangerous. There are volumes of information about raw fruits and
vegetables and their benefits for health and nutrition.

I first started studying raw nutrition in the early 1970s. One of my first books was *Juice Fasting* by Dr. Paavo Airola. Later I purchased his guidebook for health, called "How to Get Well." I also studied nutritional information by Bernard Jensen, including his book, *Blending Magic: Prize-winning Blender Recipes.* I read *Fasting Can Save Your Life* and *Fasting for Renewal of Life,* by Herbert M. Shelton, and *Living the Good Life,* by Helen and Scott Nearing. I focused on eating foods that were helpful instead of harmful, life-restoring rather than -destroying. I approached nutrition as an opportunity to offer the next generation—our children—the best materials available to them. My family history included high blood pressure and heart disease, cerebral palsy, diabetes, infertility, hair loss, emphysema, and cancer. I had childhood asthma. I just knew there had to be something I could do to ensure heath for my family. For forty years, I have studied food. For thirty of those forty years I have been a vegetarian, for ten years I have been a vegan, and for the past six years I have been primarily been eating raw. For three years, we were 100 percent raw, and we have been "high raw" (80 percent raw) ever since. As my diet evolved, my health issues disappeared. But more importantly, by studying nutrition and providing organic fruits and vegetables for my family, I feel that we have gained a level of health than few Americans enjoy these days. Learning about food is more than sensible; it is a means of survival. People who do not want you to know or learn about healthy food and nutrition are not looking out for your best interests. Michael Pollan of the *New York Times* stated: "If you're concerned about your health, you should probably avoid food products that make health claims. Why? Because a health claim on a food product is a good indication that it's not really food, and food is what you want to eat." We planted gardens, we created an organic foods co-op, we sprouted, and we grew herbs. No one quite understood what we were doing, and some were not very supportive. Others were.

WHAT I LEARNED IS NOT WHAT WE ARE TAUGHT

I learned in my studies that enzymes from raw fruits and vegetables aid in cellular healing and organ repair. When the body is not using energy to digest dense, cooked foods, it uses energy to heal. Raw foods prevent leukocytosis, or the body's defense against food as a foreign invader. Raw foods help to reverse aging by stopping inflammatory processes and encouraging healing. A raw foods diet also aids in weight loss by providing lighter foods and stopping the inflammatory process. Inflammation in the small intestine can cause Peyer's patches, which inhibit the body's ability to absorb nutrients. As a result of such inflammation, I often see children and adults who are literally living in a state of cellular starvation. We earn diseases. In America, we are led to believe that disease falls out of the sky on us. The arrogance and greed of our commercial food and medical industries encourages us to believe that we can eat and drink anything and a drug or surgery will save us from disease. The truth is that we often eat and drink our diseases into existence. We learn to avoid or dislike natural, organic raw foods that contain nutrients that are vital for our health and well-being, and we eat instead processed and harmful dead foods. If you are already eating a raw foods diet, you may be missing vital nutrients on a daily basis. My book indicates what to do to be as healthy as possible.

RAW HEALTH: AN INTRODUCTION

If you are like many people, you may take better care of your car that you do your body. You wash and wax your car, change the oil regularly, clean the interior, removing the trash, put quality gasoline in the tank, rotate the tires when needed, and get it tuned up. This machine gets us where we're going, and we don't want it to fail us or fall into disrepair. Our bodies are not made like a machine, but they get us where we're going in life and we don't want them to fail, either. While we want to look appealing on the outside to others, it isn't the $8 billion a year that women in America spend on cosmetics that make us healthy. In much the same way, it is the same for our car. We have to pay attention to what we are putting into it and cleaning out of it. This is what really counts. Just as we wouldn't put junk into our gas tank and expect positive results, we cannot put junk into our bodies and expect good performance and easy maintenance. Our bodies are living organisms that require enzymes to run well. Enzymes have been called the workhorses of the body. They make it go. We also need to attend to constant internal cleansing. We change the oil on our cars, and we need to regularly detoxify the inside of our bodies to ensure good health. Raw greens and plant fiber are magnificent detoxifiers.

Just because you have a disease or symptoms of a disease now does not mean that you have to define your life by it. In all my years as a naturopath, I have found that diseases are largely the result of poor nutrition and an accumulation of toxic substances. As we detoxify, we create a better terrain for healing to occur. In seven years, our body replaces all its cellular material. So, with some effort, you can replace dysfunctional cells with healthier cells. Most people do not know how or where to begin to heal. Drugs treat symptoms. I suggest that you follow my raw healing diet for three months to detoxify and rebuild healthier cells. Eating healthier not only can help heal, but it is a great way to prevent diseases from even beginning. You can share this method of eating with other members of your family if they are open to it. I have had mothers tell me that their teenagers healed their acne-ravaged skin, their husbands lost weight and felt an easing of their joint pain, their elderly parent's memory returned, and a vitality and passion for life was restored. In just three months. Some patients continued with eating raw and some became raw chefs and teachers. Other patients eat raw when they feel the need to get back on track or eat high raw on a daily basis.

The plan I am sharing with you does work. Just to keep it as simple as possible, I have included a one-week menu plan and grocery shopping list to get you started. There are lots of variations that you can introduce into my menu plan to change things simply by varying the types of vegetables, fruits, seeds, or nuts. I kept it very easy so that you would not feel the need for further investment in kitchen equipment. You can begin with what you have now and succeed easily. You can also purchase raw, dehydrated crackers, cookies, and bars from health food grocery stores or online. I encourage you to find a way to fill any favorite food gaps with substitutions of raw recipes online or in books dedicated to raw food preparation. I know that many patients at first miss chocolate, cookies, and salty and crunchy foods. After a week, most of these cravings pass, and you can find a substitute for almost all foods. One of my raw favorites for crunch is flax or onion crackers, but you need a dehydrator that adjusts to temperatures below 118 degrees Fahrenheit (48°C) to make them. I am sharing my recipe for easy raw cacao cookies. All it takes is dates, nuts, and cacao. Most raw food is very easy to purchase, clean, store, prepare, and enjoy.

Growing, Buying, Cleaning, and Storing Raw Produce

When it comes to fresh produce, there are degrees of freshness, and growing and picking your own produce ensures the most vibrant enzymes available. Consider growing and harvesting your own produce. I even think of sprouting as a form of gardening. You control the purchase of the organic seeds or plants; the condition of the soil that you place the seeds in, to some degree; what nutrition you feed the plants; and the natural means of dealing with weeds and pests. Produce that you pick from your own garden and eat fresh is far superior to old and prewashed, devitalized store-bought imported products. If you do not have space for a garden, or you live in the city, try container gardening. You can purchase natural, eco-friendly containers and organic soil. Our park district, located in a Chicago suburb, rents reasonably priced garden plots to residents. They till the soil in the spring, and you are notified in case you want to add fertilizer or compost to your plot. They even provide water and farm tours for you.

Buying local produce from farmers' markets or a CSA, community-supported agriculture, would be my second choice for purchasing raw fruits and vegetables. If you join a CSA, when you pick up your produce you may have the added benefit of picking additional produce that might be available. If you buy from the farmers' market, you get to know the growers and their methods firsthand. Always introduce yourself to new growers and ask them when they pick their fruit or vegetables. Try to purchase produce that was picked that morning, so the enzymes are as plentiful as possible. Confirm that their produce is organic and that no pesticides or herbicides were used on it. At our local market, one Michigan blueberry vendor was advertising "all natural" produce. When we inquired about pesticides or herbicides, the growers admitted that they sprayed the root base and rows once or twice in the early spring. *All natural* means very little, and rarely means *organic* unless it is stated specifically that it is. *Transitional* means that the growers are in the process of establishing themselves as organic, but have not yet met the standards required. Ask how far they are from being certified organic growers. Know that organic produce is not as flawless as produce that has been sprayed with pesticides. If bugs like it, your family will find it tasty, too. Getting used to the look of good organic produce is part of the educational process.

After you select your produce, you should know how to store and clean it. It's best to pick just what you need for the day if you are growing your own. You gain the largest enzyme advantage that way. If you are buying or picking in larger amounts, we find it best to store the produce in a refrigerator forty degrees Fahrenheit (4°C) or lower to prevent mold, and if you have the time to do so, only wash and prepare what you need for one meal or juicing. The produce stays fresher if you bag it and refrigerate it unwashed. Prewashed lettuce does not last long at all, and it is prewashed in chlorine (a known carcinogen) to kill bacteria. It is safer to wash the unprocessed lettuce as you get ready to use it and not ahead of time.

If we purchase lettuce, we always immediately remove and compost the outer leaves that may be contaminated by the picker or the packer. Before washing, cut the ends or roots from leafy greens like romaine or spinach. Wash your hands carefully with soap and dry them with a clean towel. Fill a large stainless steel pan with a gallon or more of water to which you have added three tablespoons (45 ml) of organic apple cider vinegar. Washing in plain water does not kill bacteria, and not washing produce before serving is, to my way of thinking, dangerous. If the lettuce is really dirty, you might rinse it before you float it in the vinegar water. Swish the leaves a few times and let it sit for about five to ten minutes to kill any bacteria. Never use the kitchen sink as a vessel to fill with water to float your lettuce. All kitchen sinks are contaminated with bacteria, from washing hands and contaminated foods to the bacteria that might form around the drain. In fact, I would recommend that you never allow any type of food to touch the inside of a kitchen sink. The sink has a previous sordid and unsavory bacterial history. Washing raw protein foods or cutlery in or near a kitchen sink adds millions of bacteria to an already unsafe area. I would also purchase a brand-new cutting board to ensure food safety. Be cautious not to let the lettuce or other produce come in contact with any physical place around the sink area.

After floating the lettuce, place it in another large stainless steel or glass bowl to rinse. I float, faucet-rinse, and inspect each leaf, if possible. I place the rinsed leaves into the strainer bowl of the salad spinner. Spinning the lettuce rids it of excess water. Tear the leaves if desired and place them in a serving bowl.

How to Wash Lettuce, Vegetables, and Fruit

1. Wash your hands with soap and water. Dry them with a clean towel.

2. Fill a stainless-steel bowl with at least 1 gallon (4 liters) of water and 3 tablespoons (45 ml) organic cider vinegar.

3. Trim off the outside leaves of purchased lettuce, if you have not done so already. Cut the ends.

4. Rinse off any dirt by running faucet water over the leaves.

5. Float lettuce leaves, or other produce or fruit, in the vinegar water for 5–10 minutes.

6. Faucet-rinse, inspect for insects, dirt, or flaws, and float the produce in a pure water–filled glass or stainless-steel bowl.

7. Strain off water from the produce; spin lettuce leaves in salad spinner. Serve.

CHAPTER 1

What to Expect on a Raw Healing Diet

If you are not your own doctor, you are a fool. Natural forces within us are the true healers of disease.

—HIPPOCRATES

Every choice you make about the food you eat each day will either contribute to your health or rob you of it. Every bite of food that you eat matters to your body. Not only should food taste good—that is a bonus—but food needs to support cellular repair and optimum health. A healing diet provides the body with the enzymes and nutrients it requires to repair cellular damage. If you flood the body with adequate amounts of enzymes from fresh fruits and vegetables, those enzymes will help your body heal. If you choose soda pop instead of pure water for drinking, your body must fight a battle with toxins rather than receive the bonus healing effects of hydrogen and oxygen.

Day after day, your body is nurtured or sabotaged by your food choices. I am grateful that you are taking the time to read this book and learn how to make informed food choices. Some chapters in my book are dedicated to information about good and bad food choices and the price that you pay for making bad choices, while others offer an outline of the raw diet program for healing. This optimum raw vegan diet is one that I have found most effective for reversing disease processes and the subsequent cellular damage inflicted on the human body by a toxic diet. If you follow this diet for only three months, you will probably lose weight and perhaps a decade of aging. I have seen it happen with every patient who has tried this diet. We will also consider the emotional aspects of food and healing. I will share a great deal of information in a very short time. Please do not feel overwhelmed by it. Keep in mind that my perspective on an ultimate diet is not the only path to wellness.

First, let me introduce myself. I am Dr. Karyn Mitchell, a naturopathic doctor with a Ph.D. in psychology. As I mentioned, for forty years I have studied psychology and emotions, diet, nutrition, and detoxification. I wanted to share this information with others who wanted to get well. That is why I became a naturopath. I really care about my patients, and I often tell them that it is not what I give them to *take* but what I encourage them to *give up* that will help their bodies heal. Not what I throw at them, but what they throw away that will restore their health and give them a better quality of life. After experiencing living foods for three months, most patients never revert to their old, destructive habits. I can help you feel better than you have in years. The information that I share on this subject can help you rid your body of toxins that feed disease and cause pain. This is a choice that only you can make. You may encounter some bumps in the road to health, but that is generally your body retracing disease processes or detoxifying. If you have any major concerns, or are already at health risk, please contact your healthiest health care provider for assistance. I also hope to assist you by providing the information in case any healing crisis might arise. A healing crisis is beneficial. Dr. Bernard Jensen once said, "Give me a healing crisis, and I can heal any disease." When you feel that you have a complete understanding of my raw foods dietary program, please feel free to share this book and information with others who are seeking a path to healing or a better quality of life.

Six years ago, our family made an important health decision to eat only raw, organic fruits and vegetables. Even though we had been vegetarian/vegan for over twenty-five years, and in extraordinarily good health, we had heard that we could lose excess body fat and reverse aging with a raw foods diet. Since it was summer and we enjoy a good salad, we decided to give it a try. We have been "hooked on raw" ever since and know that it is so much more than just salad. We have experienced the following benefits from our living foods diet with little effort:

Health: None of us has suffered illness since we changed to a raw vegan diet, and I see many sick people during the course of a week. Our immune systems seem to have achieved a new level of competency. Our muscles and joints feel much better. We experienced some detoxification, but feel much healthier because of it. We take no prescription drugs and very few supplements or vitamins. We get the nutrients we need from a varied diet of organic fruits, vegetables, and nuts. We grow what we can ourselves and buy organic locally whenever possible.

Weight loss: I have dropped two clothing sizes, and my husband now wears the same size that he wore as a senior in high school. We both feel years younger.

Energy: We have so much more energy that it is difficult to sleep more than five or six hours a night. We awaken refreshed and are more alert than ever throughout the day. We are more active than we've ever been and rarely feel tired.

Mind: My memory has improved and I am finding it easier to focus and retain what I have read. I think more clearly.

Time and space: We spend some time and effort washing, cutting, and creating our food, but there is very little to clean up afterward. There are no messy baking dishes or pots and pans to scrub. I placed a cutting board over my stove, so I have more counter space. Food preparation is simplified.

Balance: I find that I pay attention to what my body needs in terms of how much I eat and how hungry I am during the day. I have found an internal balance that has eliminated cravings. In her book, *12 Steps to End Your Addiction to Cooked Food,* raw researcher Victoria Boutenko explains: "Have you ever craved sweets? When our body needs calcium, we actually crave sweets. Calcium, in nature, has a sweet taste. If we plant strawberries in calcium rich soil, the strawberries will be very sweet . . . Soak sesame seeds and make sesame milk and drink it every day for two weeks on an empty stomach. I didn't want sweet things anymore. The balance in my body had changed."

Taste: Raw food tastes delicious. My sense of taste and smell has become more acute. I am so much more aware of the freshness of foods and can taste the difference between organic and nonorganic fruits and vegetables.

If you are interested in a raw foods diet for healing or improved health, please take time to study the various books and research on the subject. Raw food diets are very popular in California and New York. Explore gourmet meals from breakfast to dinner. You'll discover snacks, pizza, crackers, and desserts that anyone can prepare. I will share with you my top twenty favorite books (for various reasons) on the subject: *The Raw Gourmet* by Nomi Shannon, *Hooked on Raw* by Rhio, *The Raw Truth* by Jeremy A. Safron, *Sunfood Cuisine* by Frederic Patenaude, *Dining in the Raw* by Rita Ramano, *Living in the Raw* by Rose Lee Calabro, *Sunfood Diet Success System* by David Wolfe, *Raw: The Uncook Book* by Juliano Brotman, *Living Foods for Optimum Health* by Brian Clement, *Conscious Eating and the Rainbow Diet* by Gabriel Cousens, M.D., *Recipes for Longer Life* by Ann Wigmore, *Raw Food Real World* by Matthew Kenney and Sarma Melngailis, *Raw Food for Busy People* by Jordan Maerin, *Raw Food Made Easy* by Jennifer Cornbleet, *Alive in 5: Raw Gourmet Meals in Five Minutes* by Angela Elliott, *Living Cuisine* by Renee Underkoffler and Woody Harrelson, *Ani's Raw Food Kitchen* by Ani Phylo, *Rawsome* by Brigitte Mars, *Green for Life* by Victoria Boutenko, and *Rawvolution* by Matt Amsden.

From her book, *Recipes for Longer Life,* Ann Wigmore, founder of the Hippocrates Health Institute, wrote in 1986:

Living foods—sprouts, greens, wheatgrass, fresh vegetables, and fresh fruits—are the key to a healthy body and a longer, more satisfying life. They can protect us from the ravages of illness by strengthening our immunity. Biological mechanisms like the human body cannot thrive, or even survive, on synthetic processed foods and chemicals, which make up more than half of the present diet in the Western World. No amount of surgery, pills, therapy, or money can keep us well. Only a desire and willingness to learn more about nature, and to embrace her laws, can do so.

You may have the following questions and concerns whenever you engage in a healing process or a dietary change. You may ask yourself, "Where and how do I begin? Or what can I expect during this process?" Hopefully, this will all be explained to you, but I want you to know right away what good things that might be in store for you:

1. Rejuvenation: reversing the aging process
   - hair and skin becoming more radiant
   - less sleep required; more energy throughout the day
   - greater joint flexibility and less pain
   - pancreas may shrink

- improvement in vision
- disease processes may heal
- easier digestion and better bowel and elimination processes

2. Weight loss: Cravings disappear (cravings for sugars and starches, in particular)

3. More vitality, health, and passion for life.

I know that you have heard that it is not the quantity of life that you live but the quality of life that you enjoy that makes life worth living. You can choose to live a pain- and disease-free, youthful life. It is all about your choices. Love yourself enough to make good choices about what you eat each and every day. Everything that you choose to eat either contributes to wellness and energy or deprives you of them. From an early age, everything that you consumed created the body that you live in now. Since you have the miraculous potential to create an entire new cellular body every seven years, choosing to eat raw, organic, nutrient-rich foods can contribute to a level of wellness that you never imagined you could achieve.

Whether you are facing a life-threatening illness or wish to reverse aging, a raw nutritional diet plan is a simple three-month program that will help you to heal and feel better. If you have never before detoxified your body with enzyme-rich, living foods, now is a great time to begin. Of all of the detoxification regimens, consuming raw, plant-based foods is one of the most productive and simplest of all. You will be amazed at the results. You can effortlessly lose weight if that is your goal, and most people look and feel ten years younger in just three months. After that time, you may wish to follow a more general raw diet or incorporate more raw foods into your more conscious eating plan. If you want to be active, pain-free, and healthy, you need to study nutrition and invest in a more conscious way of eating. You have to change your old eating habits.

The Courage to Change Your Old Pattern of Eating

Changing your diet may make you feel as if you are changing who you are. For some, it may feel scary; to others, exciting. If you change your diet, you are embarking on a new life. Anthropologist Victor Turner described such a change or initiation as the "time between no longer and not yet." It seems like a scary place because we cannot control it.

There are three stages to this process: separation, transition, and reincorporation.

1. Separation
   - Recognizing that change is necessary
   - Finding the will or force to change
   - Initiating the needed change
   - Working through any resistance

2. Transition
   - Engaging the process of change
   - Getting comfortable with a new way of being and feeling
   - Finding yourself in the uncertain free fall of betwixt and between
   - Deconstructing old patterns
   - Defining your new self

3. Reincorporation
   - Establishing a new norm through rebuilding
   - Finding strength and stability in the new lifestyle
   - Transforming and healing the physical, mental, emotional, and spiritual dimensions
   - Creating a new and healthier life

Change is not always easy, but knowing that you have the courage to change is transformative. A life-threatening disease forces us to change old habits. A patient of mine shared his experience with a life-threatening cancer:

When my wife heard the diagnosis, she got this determined look in her eyes. She set up flowcharts for my drugs, surgeries, chemotherapy treatments, and trips to the oncologist. As a businesswoman, she was managing my "cancer account" in the only way she knew how. When I refused the final horrendous surgery that might possibly "save my life," my wife was incredulous. I told her that I couldn't and wouldn't live with the consequences of that surgery. I'd rather die. I had been researching holistic methods of treating cancer. I told her I wanted to try herbs and raw foods, fasting and juicing, and reiki. When the oncologist washed his hands of me, that is when I lost my wife. I knew that, for whatever reason, she had invested herself 100 percent in the cut, slash, and burn treatments. I tried to talk to her, to get her to understand how I felt about being gutted, but I knew that this was no longer about me. It was about her finding a new purpose in life. She felt needed when I was too sick to hold my head up after chemotherapy. She soaked up the sympathy that she got from her friends and the doctors and nurses. I was so grateful for all that she did for me. I expressed it often. But she couldn't seem to really connect with the pain that I suffered during the horrible treatments and surgeries. She just couldn't deal with me finding a way outside the hospital setting to get well. She told me that she was embarrassed by my actions. But I have to tell you, I am convinced that the only reason that I am alive today, many years later, is because I had the courage to look outside the box and take responsibility for my own healing. I had to make the changes to live in spite of the loss of my support system.

The experience described above illustrates all those scary stages of change. Deepak Chopra refers to what others have called *quantum healing*. He says that you must clarify your intended outcome and set its intention in your consciousness. It seems that our DNA may be programmable and is far more responsive and interactive with our brain than we realize. So the process of change—separation, transition, and reincorporation—may reset or reprogram the dynamic of healing within the mind and physical body. When you heal from such an incurable disease, it seems like a miracle, but perhaps it is as simple as embracing that intention to heal and accepting the responsibility to change old habits. That step may unleash the possibilities, power, and potential that lie deep within you.

DO STOMACH ACIDS DESTROY ENZYMES?

One question that people often ask about eating an enzyme-rich raw diet is if the acids present in the stomach don't destroy them before they are used by the body. Enzyme researcher Viktoras Kulvinska proved that stomach acid merely deactivates food enzymes. These are then reactivated when they are in the more alkaline environment of the small intestine. People who switch to a raw vegan diet are free of cooked protein foods, which require large secretions of stomach acid.

Dr. Edward Howell, M.D., further clarifies for us how enzymes work in the gut:

Although nutritionists claim that enzymes in food are destroyed in the stomach, they overlook two important facts. First of all, when you eat food, acid secretion is minimal for at least thirty minutes. As the food goes down the esophagus, it drops into the top portion of the stomach. This is called the cardiac section, since it is closer to the heart. The bottom part of the stomach (the pyloric) remains flat and closed while the cardiac section opens up to accommodate the food. During the time the food sits in the upper section, very few enzymes are secreted by the body. The enzymes in the food itself go about digesting the food. The more of this self-digestion that occurs, the less work the body has to do later. When this thirty- to forty-five-minute period is over, the bottom section of the stomach opens up and the body starts secreting acid and enzymes. Even at this point, the food enzymes are not inactivated until the acid level becomes more prohibitive. You see, food enzymes can tolerate chemical environments many times more acid than neutral.

Enzymes are substances which make life possible. They are needed for every chemical reaction in that occurs in our body. Without enzymes, no activity at all would take place. Vitamins, minerals, and hormones cannot do any work without enzymes. We inherit a certain enzyme potential at birth. This limited supply of activity factors or life force must last us a lifetime. It's just as if you inherited a certain amount of money. If the movement is all one way—all spending and no income—you will run out of money. Likewise, the faster you use up your supply of enzyme activity, the quicker you will run out. Just about every single person eats a diet of mainly cooked foods. Keep in mind that whenever a food is boiled at 212 degrees [100°C], the enzymes in it are 100 percent destroyed. If enzymes were in the food we eat, they would do some or even a considerable part of the work of digestion by themselves. However, when you eat cooked, enzyme-free food, this forces the body itself to make the enzymes needed for digestion. A diet that consists of mostly cooked food is one of the paramount causes of premature aging and early death. I also believe it's the underlying cause of almost all degenerative diseases. If the body is overburdened to supply many enzymes to the saliva, gastric juice, pancreatic juice, and intestinal juice, then it must curtail the production of enzymes for other purposes. If this occurs, then how can the body also make enough enzymes to run the brain, heart, kidneys, lungs, muscles, and other organs and tissues? The body steals enzymes from richer sources. This "stealing" of enzymes from other parts of the body to service the digestive tract sets up a competition for enzymes among the various organ systems and tissues of the body. The resulting metabolic dislocations may be the direct cause of cancer, coronary heart disease, diabetes, and many other chronic incurable diseases. This state of enzyme deficiency stress exists in the majority of persons on the civilized, enzyme-free diet. There is evidence that rats on a cooked diet have a pancreas about twice as heavy as rats on a raw diet. Moreover, evidence shows that the human pancreas is one of the heaviest in the animal kingdom, when you adjust for total body weight. This over-enlargement of the human pancreas is just as dangerous—probably even more so—than an over-enlargement of the heart, the thyroid, and so on. The overproduction of enzymes in humans is a pathological adaption to a diet of enzyme-free foods. The pancreas is not the only part of the body that over-secretes enzymes when the diet is cooked. In addition, there are the human salivary glands, which produce enzymes to a degree never found in wild animals on their natural foods. Another effect associated with food enzyme deficiency is that the size of the brain decreases. In addition, the thyroid over-enlarges, even in the presence of adequate iodine. This has been shown in a number of species. From my work in a sanitarium many years ago, I've found that it was impossible to get people fat on raw foods, regardless of the calorie intake. Humans could expand their lives by twenty years just by consuming adequate enzymes. Other things being equal, you live as long as your body has enzyme activity factors to make enzymes from. When it gets to the point that you can't make certain enzymes, then your life ends. Enzymes may be the key factor in preventing chronic disease and extending the human lifespan.

Dr. Howell began his study of food enzymes and human health more than fifty years ago. He is the author of *The Status of Food Enzymes in Digestion and Metabolism* and *Enzyme Nutrition*. His books are an invaluable resource for enzyme information.

CHAPTER 2

Our Illusion of Health: We May Look Good on Paper

More die in the United States of too much food than of too little.
—JOHN KENNETH GALBRAITH, *THE AFFLUENT SOCIETY*

When I interview new patients for the first time, I always ask them how they would rate their health. Most of them will relate to me that they feel they are in good or excellent health because they have a regular bowel movement once a week and only get sick one or two times a year. This is what I call the "illusion of health," which actually prevents us from achieving true wellness. The wellness bar in this country is set pretty low when compared to other countries. Other countries focus on vital nutrition and organic foods and take food seriously, eating their food slowly and consciously. Foods prevent disease.

There are levels to health that are directly related to emotional and mental well-being. That being said, there are also levels to disease that are directly related to the inability to make good choices related to health. I believe that there is a direct correlation between the ability to make good food choices when you are well and a compromised ability to make good food choices when you are sick. In that respect, I often find that new patients who come to me when they are already fighting a disease process are rarely open to a new way of thinking about food. That is why I spend so much time educating new patients about reversing their disease with enzyme-rich raw foods. It is not difficult to remember what is on the list or off it. Raw foods are fruits and vegetables that do not come prepackaged in a can or bottle. You can imagine how sad it was for our raw foods group when a young mother came to her first

16

(and last) raw potluck with a bag of old apples and a tab-pull can of processed caramel. Mom had carried along a baggie of fruit loops for her baby to chew on. Most people never have the opportunity to learn what good foods are or how good you feel when you eat an enzyme-rich diet. The dark shadow that is cast by sugary, white, acidic foods is a long one. Acidic foods cause intense cravings. And when you are not physically, mentally, or emotionally well enough to fight for wellness, the disease often wins. This negative cycle of feeding the sugar and yeast dragon within often keeps the mind in an unstable state. It is hard to think straight through the haze of brain fog that yeasty beasties create.

There are many concerns that we might have about our current level of health in America. Since I have been alive for over a half a century, I have observed that you cannot go anywhere without seeing sick or obese children, or dine without overhearing conversations about someone's chemotherapy treatments or surgeries. We consider all this as normal now, and I think it is such complacency that keeps us from being shocked about the degradation of health here. Cancer rates are approaching one in two, and childhood diabetes and immune diseases like fibromyalgia are on the rise. I find such statistics scary, and what I hear and don't hear, and see and don't see, in our country even more so. We should be outraged that we are ranked number one in health care costs: insurance per year per person in this country costs an average of over $8,000. That was my entire salary in my first year of teaching. You would think that this would ensure us the best health care in the world, yet the United States ranks at the very bottom of all industrialized countries in quality of health care, while our health care costs are eight times that of the next to the last nation. We are the only industrialized nation without universal health care. For the most part, Americans are kept in the dark about their anatomy or the most elemental nutritional requirements of the body. We are led to believe that our body is like a foreign car that depends on a mechanic far more intelligent than we are to maintain it. On the other hand, we are sold the most inefficient and damaging fuels to run it. But the truth is, our bodies are not cars, nor are they made of nonorganic compounds. Yet every time we turn around, some FDA-approved plastic or nonorganic drug or food is "approved" for our use. We have to be savvy consumers to protect our biological health. In order for us to be healthy, we have to eat healthy, organic, fresh foods. We must learn to care for ourselves. We must learn what real, nutritious food is and avoid processed junk food.

Research published in March 2010 in the journal *Neuroscience* revealed just how addictive junk food can be. Rats were offered unlimited access to a diet of bacon, pound cake, candy bars, and other junk food. They gained lots of weight. Even as they grew fatter, the rats kept eating as if they were compelled to do so. They were even given unpleasant shocks to their feet to discourage them from eating, but they could not stop eating. Meanwhile, another group of rats were fed a well-balanced, healthy diet and only given limited access to junk food. They did not gain much weight and stopped eating immediately when a shock cue was imminent. An even more startling finding was that when researchers took the junk food away from the obese rats and replaced it with healthy food, the obese rats refused to eat almost anything for two weeks. Speaking about this ignored response by the obese rats, Paul Kenny, an associate professor at Scripps Research Institute in Jupiter, Florida, said, "They went into voluntary starvation. Researchers feel that this might translate into an ominous warning for human behavior. It is possible that a diet heavy in junk and processed foods might cause changes in the brain. When the brain goes awry, the result is not only that people gain weight, but that they feel compelled to seek out more and more junk food." When researchers looked at the obese rats' brains, they found a decline in the dopamine D2 receptor that recent research has implicated in addiction to cocaine and heroine. Kenny remarked that "A hallmark of drug addiction is that it leads to changes in how the brain's reward system works. *Addiction* is a loaded term, but in this case, there is evidence of addictive adaptations. What we think is happening is that, as you become obese over a period of time, the dopamine D2 receptors go down, which plays a role in becoming a compulsive eater."

Pietro Cottone, assistant professor of addictive disorders at Boston University School of Medicine, states that "There could also be something in the accumulated fat itself that alters the brain's reward threshold, setting up a vicious cycle of overeating yet not feeling satisfied. The only way to return to normality is probably dieting for a long period of time to lose the body weight and not eating junk food. The withdrawal effects in the brain may be the same as withdrawing from drugs and alcohol."

When I teach classes about the immune system, I point out that practitioners of allopathic (Western) medicine have no idea what or where the immune system actually is. Why is it misunderstood and misplaced like an old brown shoe in a closet? Because it transcends the technological, mechanistic medical model of what the body is. The body as viewed as a machine has no innate defense mechanisms, so a false defense system must be created for it. The mistake in this type of thinking has led us down some dangerous paths. It may surprise you to know that our so-called "health care system" is not about health at all. It has become a "disease care system." I have spent decades researching cancer and autoimmune disorders and have come to the conclusion that you cannot depend on any government or health care agency in this country to give you the truth about how to get or stay well. I have decided that if government officials even have a clue as to how that might be done, they are certainly keeping it a secret from the rest of the population. Our bodies are created from the genetic material of our ancestors, their toxic load included. We also build our biological bodies daily with junk or good enzyme-rich foods that we eat. We also pollute our bodies with nonbiological, chemical substances, such as trans fats, pharmaceutical drugs, and excessive vaccines, as well as polluted water and air. If we eat well, our body will be much better equipped to deal with the toxins present in our environment.

Bad food choices also lower your immune reservoir. Diseases, surgeries, and drugs lower your immune reservoir. Unfortunately, every child born to a mother who has a compromised immune system not only has a diminished chance for health, but that firstborn child downloads the mother's toxic burden. Research done by Stanford Hospital on the cord blood of newborn children revealed that, on average, every newborn's blood contains over two hundred hazardous toxic chemicals. When we think of health, we cannot ignore the immune system. Enzymes in our food offer us the opportunity to reverse some, if not most, of the damage done by our poor eating habits. It takes time. And with other naturopathic and biological efforts, we can reverse some of the other types of damage as well. We are biological creatures, not machines. We need to live in a healthy environment and eat well if we want to live a long, healthy, pain-free life. The mammalian formula for life expectancy is ten times our age at puberty. Most humans are not living half that long because we have forgotten our true diet and lifestyle. In her book *Edible Medicines*, Nina L. Etkins, former professor of medical anthropology at the University of Hawaii, states:

> Foods and food processing in contemporary affluent populations include a vast array of commercially produced items whose natural origins are ambiguous. Despite the increased diversity of products available, those consumed in highest proportion contain high concentrations of sugar or

sweeteners, salt, fats, and refined grains. A vast literature—both scientific and popular—records the complex relationships of these dietary excesses to hypertension, obesity, elevated cholesterol, cardiovascular diseases, and cancers. The quality of contemporary diets is further compromised by diminished fruit, vegetable, and fiber intake and by sedentary lifestyles. Among affluent populations in the West, and increasingly elsewhere, there is a growing apprehension of these insalubrious consequences of long-term nutrition transition.

National Geographic magazine writer Dan Buettner shared his research on longevity in his book called *The Blue Zones: Lessons for Living Longer from the People Who've Lived the Longest.* Four "Blue Zones" of longevity have been identified in the world. These are: Okinawa, Japan; Sardinia, Italy; Nicoya Peninsula, Costa Rica; and Loma Linda, California, where there is a large population of Seventh-Day Adventists who maintain a strict vegetarian diet. The individuals who live in these Blue Zones have more people who have lived over the age of one hundred, and a higher chance of reaching a healthy age of ninety, than anywhere else on earth. What Buettner discovered in his research are nine common elements. Residents of these areas:

1. Cut calories
2. Avoid meat and processed foods
3. Move naturally
4. Maintain a positive outlook on life
5. Keep their stress levels low
6. Put family first
7. Belong to a community
8. Drink alcohol (especially red wine) in extreme moderation
9. Surround themselves with people who have similar Blue Zone values.

Scientists have concluded that less than 25 percent of longevity is determined by our ancestors' genes. The remaining 75 percent depends directly on our lifestyle and dietary choices. The best advice, particularly in the controversial world of nutrition and diet, is simple: A plant-based diet is an essential part of any healthful nutritional program. There is overwhelming evidence from the four Blue Zones confirming that the regular consumption of vegetables and fruits promotes longevity. You might note that you don't have to be completely vegetarian to do this. Not everyone living long and healthy lives in the four Blue Zones is vegetarian, but their primary diet is plant-based and junk-free.

We recently had the opportunity to visit Costa Rica and learned a great deal about why a Blue Zone might be located there. I always pay attention to what people are eating when they are in restaurants. For lunch, many of the locals were eating salads and fresh, locally grown fruit. There was very little beef eaten, since it was imported from Brazil for the most part. The local supermarkets were filled with fresh fruits and vegetables. One grocery store targeting tourist dollars in the town of Jaco advertised that they had "aisles of American junk food." Americans do go to Costa Rica for their cheaper medical, dental, and surgical procedures. Cosmetic surgery, in particular, is an attraction. When I was observing people, it seemed to me that the only overweight and obviously unhealthy people in Costa Rica were Americans. I spoke to a local guide about Costa Rican health. What he said was, "Americans are sick because they eat sick food. Most of us here only eat healthy food. Loving mommas don't let their babies eat sick food." In the dedication to his book *Blending Magic,* which he wrote in 1954, Dr. Bernard Jensen stated:

> This book is dedicated to those housewives who are seeking, finding, and using the finest equipment (blenders) and the finest foods in their kitchen to keep their family in the best of health. Into their hands I pray and hope that the finest knowledge and information be given that those who are depending on her for their health may know what it is to really "feel wonderful."

In that same book, he explains why liquefied foods are important:

> Americans generally buy foods grown in impoverished soil, and they must make up in bulk for the below-standard foods they consume. For example, a carrot grown in Sweden will probably be ten times more nutritious than a carrot grown on one of the big forced-production farms in the California Imperial Valley. The Swedish carrot may be smaller, but it will have less water and more vitamins, consequently being of more value from a nutritional standpoint. In many cases, the American carrot is grown with chemical fertilizers and is forced to mature quickly. The real

crux of the problem is that our food can be no better than the soil from
which it springs. Inferior soil produces inferior food. Soil that does not
have the proper minerals and the other factors needed for healthy plant
life is not going to produce healthy fruits and vegetables.

While "housewives" are an endangered species, someone needs to foster
good eating habits. It has been proven that children need to sit down with
adults for at least one meal—any meal—a day. Whether it is Mom, Dad,
Grandma, or Grandpa doesn't matter as long as someone cares enough to provide food to meet children's basic needs. The foraging generation of children is
failing to thrive, and many of them are clinically depressed and unable to
reproduce. No wonder. They eat sick food and, consequently, they get sick.

Medical schools perpetuate the illusion of health by failing to provide good
nutrition training for aspiring doctors. It is estimated that of the 125 medical
schools in the United States, only 30 of them require their students to take a
single course in nutrition. The average number of hours invested in nutrition
education for the average American physician during four years of school is
$2^{1}/_{2}$ hours. Since that is the case, doctors are ill-equipped to give nutritional
advice or implement educational programs for health, even though most modern illnesses are food and lifestyle induced. While more and more studies confirm the link between food choices and disease prevention, medical school
curricula continue to focus on and invest in drug-dispensing practices as a
means of suppressing illness and offering a quick fix that gives patients immediate gratification but may cause more harm in the long term. In the meantime,
the concept of actually preventing the alarming rise of newly diagnosed cases
of cancer, heart disease, autism, and diabetes by cultivating good nutritional
choices is ignored and downplayed. Most doctors are afraid to discuss nutrition with patients because they know absolutely nothing about it and fail to
understand the importance of it in preventing or reversing disease processes.
Mike Adams,writing on the site naturalnews.com, is blunt:

The future of medicine is in true healing. And I believe that in the future,
people will look back at the time period we're in right now and be
amazed. They'll say, "How could these people have just poisoned the
entire population with chemicals, and even advertised them on TV!? How
could people even call themselves doctors when all they did was write
prescription drugs for people? They're just drug dealers. How dare they

even call themselves doctors? And how could the medical schools not even teach nutrition? How could it be?!" Foods and nutrition are the foundation of health, yet doctors are being given virtually no education whatsoever in this area.

After his second diagnosis of a brain tumor, Dr. David Servan-Schreiber, a founding member of Doctors Without Borders, stated in the April 2009 issue of *Psychology Today:*

When doctors say it doesn't matter what you eat, I knew they didn't know. I'd given this stock answer to people myself, not knowing what I was saying. Nobody invites physicians to a course on the benefits of yoga, jogging, broccoli, and garlic. Physicians do very little to help your body do its part to fight disease. They target the tumor but don't support the terrain. People need to know they can go further. Physicians believe that most people do not want to change. But certainly I was quite willing to change. It's hard for me to imagine I'm the only one. One hundred percent of people have cancer cells in their bodies after the age of fifty.

In natural medicine, we know that if we feed those latent cancer cells sugar and toxic substances, we create further illness. If we limit, inhibit, or eliminate them with diet, exercise, and detoxification efforts, we can bring about wellness. If a patient asks a question about the link between disease and nutrition, her doctor will ignore the question or perhaps refer her to a nutritionist for nutritional counseling. The unfortunate result of this referral is that nutrition schools are often funded by commercial food industries, like the dairy industry, the fake sugar industry, or green gelatin hospital foods. By contrast, most traditional naturopathic doctors spend the majority of their formal educational training studying how to heal the body through nutrition. Even in core courses of phytopharmacology, the nutritional and chemical aspects of plants are studied. There is little interest in commercial funding for most traditional naturopathic education, since these doctors do not accept the financial support of any commercial purveyors of toxic foods or drugs. A health consumer must be savvy in finding his way through America's big industrial medical market. Our economy has been rightfully labeled a "medical-industrial complex." The latest moneymaking trend is for allopathic doctors to pretend to be educated or interested in "natural" or "holistic" or "complementary" medicine. This means patients are advised to spend massive amounts of dollars for the most expensive vitamin supplements in addition to the usual prescriptions for drugs or antibiotics. Because they are not well educated, these supplements contain cheap fillers that tax the kidneys. Pharmaceutical drugs can cause debilitating nutritional deficiencies. I have often encountered patients who were taking nearly a dozen pharmaceutical drugs who were suffering such severe nutritional deficiencies that they were malnourished. One woman in her late eighties looked like she was starving to death. Her ribs were protruding, she was underweight, the whites of her eyes were yellow, and mucus poured from her nose. She could hardly hold her head up, and both her thinking and speech were unclear. She was taking forty-two prescription drugs daily. Her nutritional blood tests indicated that she had a severe deficiency in most vitamins, especially vitamins A, C, B_6, B_{12}, and D. Due to drug-induced nutritional deficiencies and subsequent malabsorption, her body was unable to absorb vitamins from her food. She was very depressed and angry, even though she was on two antidepressants. Research indicates that B_6 depletion can cause depression. She is now ninety-two and free of all pharmaceutical drugs. Her diet is good, her eyes shine, and she has few age spots on her face and hands. She looks like she is seventy, and is a very different person than when I first met her. She can hold her head up, she smiles, and she is rarely depressed.

In the book *Drug Induced Nutritional Deficiencies,* by Daphne A. Roe, M.D., the following information is shared:

> If no specific etiology for anemia can be determined, it is frequently labeled as a "nutritional anemia," with little thought given to its pathogenesis or treatment. Much of the thinking we do about the nutrition of patients is superficial, largely because our education in this subject has also been superficial. Many medical schools treat the subject with disdain. Nutrition is considered appropriate material for nurses and dieticians, but not for medical students. In addition to influencing dietary intake, drugs affect the metabolism of nutrients at a wide variety of sites, including intestinal absorption, plasma-binding and transport, peripheral utilization, transport across cell membranes, intracellular reactions, storage in tissues, turnover, and elimination and excretion. It is evident that drugs are important causes of malnutrition, in addition to their other side effects. This problem must be considered particularly with respect to older individuals who constitute the largest group of drug users.

Your quality of life depends on what you eat and what you don't take as drugs; you can nurture yourself properly with good food. Years ago, when I read *Coyote Medicine,* by Lewis Mehl-Madrona, M.D., I identified with his sense of disillusionment with allopathic medicine: "I thought that other doctors shared my own ideal of medicine: that its purpose was to restore unwell persons to health. Imagine my surprise on hearing a renowned professor of internal medicine begin a lecture by noting that the physician's job lay in 'slowing and making less painful the patient's inexorable and inevitable progression toward death and decay.' "

I will never forget the Thanksgiving gathering that our family had in a hospital in Iowa City. My ninety-five-year-old father-in-law was in recovery from a surgery for an iatrogenic (doctor- and drug-induced) event. The surgeon took a few moments to assure us that my father-in-law was doing well, and a new drug was being added to a long list of others. I was concerned about the horrible diet they had been feeding him while he was in the hospital. I wasn't so certain that his digestive system or his heart could survive all the beef, ham, potatoes, noodles, and Honduran sugar–packed fruit and cakes they were serving there. I asked if his diet could be healthier and heart smart. The surgeon gave me a condescending look and replied, "Miss, let the man eat what he wants! He's ninety-five years old. If he was younger, it might matter." I told him that I respectfully disagreed with him and that his wife was very careful what she fed him at home. His food was very carefully selected and prepared because we all wanted him around for a while longer. He shrugged as he left and said, "It doesn't matter."

I'm telling you that what you eat each and every day *does* matter. The surgeon's message was clear: good nutrition doesn't matter. Just because most medical doctors ignore nutrition, because they neglected to learn about it, doesn't mean that it doesn't matter. They cut themselves off from what they do not know. They are uncomfortable with what they do not know.

CHAPTER 3

Plants Provide More Than Adequate Vitamins and Nutrients

*The world is biologically complex: no organism can
be understood outside the context of its place in nature
and the other organisms that share that environment.*

—NINA L. ETKINS, *EDIBLE MEDICINES:
AN ETHNOPHARMACOLOGY OF FOOD*

According to the U.S. Department of Agriculture nutrient database, a few foods were analyzed for their vitamin levels in raw versus cooked varieties. The results of this study were fascinating, as noted in Table 3-1.

TABLE 3-1	VITAMINS LOST IN BOILING, PER 100 GRAMS OF FOOD					
VITAMIN ASSAY	C	B_1	B_2	B_3	B_5	B_6
Broccoli, raw	93	.065	.12	.64	.53	.16
Broccoli, boiled	75	.055	.11	.57	.51	.14
Carrots, raw	9.3	.097	.059	.93	.20	.15
Carrots, boiled	2.3	.034	.056	.51	.30	.25

Across the board, most cooked vegetable suffered a loss of nutrients. The USDA concluded: "Average vitamin losses after correction for water loss range from about 10 to 25 percent in most cases."

If we need vitamins and minerals, and soil depletion makes our foods less nutritious than those consumed by generations past, it makes sense to eat raw fruits and vegetables, grown locally.

26

Table 3-2 spells out the Council for Responsible Nutrition's recommended daily consumption of vitamins and minerals.

TABLE 3-2	VITAMIN AND MINERAL RECOMMENDATIONS	
VITAMIN	CURRENT RDI*	NEW DRI**
Vitamin A	5,000 International Units (IU)	900 micrograms (mcg); (3,000 IU)
Vitamin C	60 milligrams (mg)	90 mg
Vitamin D	400 IU (10 mcg)	15 mcg (600 IU)
Vitamin E	30 IU (20 mg)	15 mg
Vitamin K	80 mcg	120 mcg
Thiamine	1.5 mg	1.2 mg
Riboflavin	1.7 mg	1.3 mg
Niacin	20 mg	16 mg
Vitamin B_6	2 mg	1.7 mg
Folate	400 mcg (0.4 mg)	400 mcg from food; 200 mcg, synthetic
Vitamin B_{12}	6 mcg	2.4 mcg
Biotin	300 mcg	30 mcg
Pantothenic acid	10 mg	5 mg
Choline	Not established	550 mg

*The Reference Daily Intake (RDI) is the value established by the Food and Drug Administration (FDA) for use in nutrition labeling. It was based initially on the highest 1968 Recommended Dietary Allowance (RDA) for each nutrient to ensure that needs were met for all age groups.

**The Dietary Reference Intakes (DRI) is the most recent set of dietary recommendations established by the Food and Nutrition Board of the Institute of Medicine, 1997–2001. They replace previous RDAs.

USDA Table of Nutrient Retention Factors (2003).

According to Mayo Clinic research:

The fact of the matter is that a very large number of people don't get all of the nutrients their body needs from their diet because they either can't or don't eat enough, or they can't or don't eat a large variety of healthy foods. Whole foods contain nutrients and dietary fiber that are believed to be important for good health and proper digestion. Whole foods may also help to prevent a variety of common, yet deadly diseases including cancer, heart disease, and diabetes. Whole foods are complex. They contain a large variety and unique mixture of the micronutrients your body requires—not just one or two. An orange you buy at the local supermarket, for example, provides not only vitamin C but also calcium, beta-carotene, and other important nutrients. A vitamin C supplement alone cannot supply the body with these other micronutrients gained by eating a simple orange. Sufficient fiber intake also helps prevent constipation. Most experts agree that whole foods are the best sources of the vitamins and minerals the body requires to stay healthy and fit. Both minerals and vitamins are substances your body requires in small but regular amounts for proper growth, health, and body function. Together, vitamins and minerals are referred to as micronutrients. The human body is not capable of producing micronutrients, so you must get them from the foods you eat or from dietary supplements. Vitamins are necessary for a plethora of biologic processes in the body, including digestion, growth, alertness and the ability to fight infection. They also make it possible for your body to process and use proteins, nutrients and fats. Vitamins also act as catalysts—responsible for initiating or increasing chemical reactions.

Water-soluble vitamins including Vitamin C, biotin and the seven other B vitamins—thiamine (B_1), riboflavin (B_2), niacin (B_3), pantothenic acid (B_5), pyridoxine (B_6), folic acid (B_9) and cobalamin (B_{12})—dissolve in water (water-soluble) and aren't stored in your body in any significant amounts. Water-soluble vitamins that are not immediately used by the body are simply excreted in body by urine.

Fat-soluble vitamins including A, D, E or K, unlike water-soluble vitamins, when not used by the body right after ingestion are stored as body fat and in the liver. When taken in excess, fat-soluble vitamins can accumulate in the human body and eventually become toxic. The body is especially sensitive to excessive amounts of vitamins D and A. And since vitamins E and K affect blood clotting, it is highly recommended that you talk with a doctor before taking a vitamin or mineral supplement as it thins the blood if you are taking a drug like Warfarin.

Minerals are the primary components in your bones and teeth, and they are also the building blocks for other cells and enzymes found throughout the human body. Minerals assist in regulating the balance of fluids in the body and affect the movement of nerve impulses. There are even some minerals that help carry much-needed oxygen to cells and carry away harmful carbon dioxide. There are two classes of mineral: major minerals and trace minerals. Major minerals include calcium, phosphorus, magnesium, potassium, sodium, sulfur and chloride. They are classified as major minerals because most adults require these minerals in relatively large amounts—that is, more than 250 milligrams (mg) a day. Trace minerals include chromium, copper, fluoride, iron, iodine, manganese, molybdenum, selenium and zinc. They are classified as trace minerals because the human body requires them in smaller amounts—less than 20 mg a day.

Eleven of our thirteen essential vitamins come directly from plants. Vitamin D comes from sunlight, but in certain parts of the world, sunlight is not available enough to be considered useful. Vitamin D, like the other fat-soluble vitamins A, E, and K, is stored in the tissues for long periods. B_{12} is available from nutritional yeast or fermented, plant-based foods. Plant foods created by complex biological processes are the most abundant sources of nutrition on earth, according to Nina L. Etkins, as noted in her book, *Edible Medicines:*

Plants assimilate simple substances such as mineral and atmospheric gases and synthesize the complex organic molecules necessary for reproduction, growth, and differentiation into specialized tissues and organs. Most plant physiology is mediated by biochemical pathways that are functionally distinguished as primary or secondary. Primary metabolism is consider essential to normal cellular function, for example, biochemical pathways involved in its respiration, the oxidation of carbohydrates to provide energy, water, and carbon dioxide; photosynthesis is the use of chlorophyll and solar energy to produce carbohydrates.

In spite of what you've been told by food industry lobbies and various interest groups, animal foods are not essential forms of vitamins, protein, calcium, amino acids, or essential fats. Most heart-protecting, cancer-fighting, and immune-enhancing substances come from the phytochemicals in plants. If you want to get well and stay well, you have to keep this in mind. Antioxidant vitamins C and E, plus beta-carotene and other health-promoting substances, come from plants. Plants also contain fiber, one of the main substances that protect us from cancers, primarily of the large intestine and breast. All the protein you need can be easily obtained by consuming plant foods alone. These plant foods contain complete proteins and amino acids. Most Americans are eating ten times more protein than they need, and most of it is animal-based protein, which may cause cancer because it lacks fiber. Animal-based protein is also very challenging to the liver and kidneys. If what you are eating every day is making you sick, if you feel that you have no energy, and if you have been diagnosed with a disease or health concern of any kind, I urge you to change to a raw diet for at least three months. My nutritional 4-3-2-1 Raw Healing Diet Plan should be called "4-3-2-1 for 3." In only three months you should feel like a younger, healthier person. If you get frustrated or angry about a change from what has been making you sick, then you have to know deep inside that perhaps you have an emotional addiction to acidic foods as well, especially foods like meat and sugar. See Chapter 4 for more information concerning emotional food addiction.

Navigating the USDA website is difficult because it is inundated with information from interest groups. One of the databases illustrates how many nutrients in vegetables are lost during cooking. The specific type of "cooking" that is considered seems to be missing from the site and should be considered, to my way of thinking. Further scientific analysis shows that too much heat and water during the process of cooking vegetables can cause the loss of phytochemicals, vitamins, and minerals. The key to retaining the nutrients in vegetables would be to eat them raw and in their natural state. Otherwise, research indicates that if you do cook vegetables, to preserve their nutrients, cook them quickly and with little water, or stir-fry them in healthful oil, such as olive oil or another monounsaturated oil. Boiling vegetables in a pan of water leads to loss of water-soluble vitamins like vitamin C and folate, an important B vitamin.

Studies show that certain antioxidant, cancer-fighting phytochemicals are also lost in the cooking water. Lost are the antioxidants called glucosinolates in broccoli and other cruciferous vegetables. When comparing boiled to steamed broccoli, analysis found that steamed broccoli contained less vitamin C and glucosinolates than raw broccoli, but more than boiled broccoli. Boiling broccoli and spinach can cause a 50 percent loss of folate.

Zucchini, beans, and carrots, cooked in little water, are significantly higher in phytochemicals called flavonoids than those cooked in larger amounts of water. Cruciferous vegetables, including broccoli, Brussels sprouts, and cabbage, lose about 90 percent of their glucosinolates when boiled, but show no significant loss when steamed or stir-fried.

A quick cooking time seems to minimize the loss of heat-sensitive vitamins, such as vitamins C and B. Oven roasting is another way to cook vegetables without immersing them in water. But when cooked at higher temperatures for longer periods—often thirty to forty minutes at four hundred degrees (204°C)—vegetables may lose nutrients when compared to other water-free cooking methods. Again, you lose enzymes when you cook vegetables, and you lose phytonutrients. Why cook away the food value?

Another fact to consider is that our current soils are so polluted and depleted that we cannot look back to our grandparents or even our parents and claim that longevity is on our side. Our foodless foods have created unhealthy cellular anomalies that diminish the health of the population with each subsequent generation. I recently came across a fact that shocked me: In 1914, an apple contained almost half the daily requirements of iron, but today you would have to eat twenty-six apples to get the same amount. In eighty years, apples have declined in nutritional value to the following extent: calcium, 48 percent; phosphorus, 84 percent; iron, 96 percent; and magnesium, the heart-helping nutrient, has dropped 82 percent. The amount of calcium in vegetables has also declined: 81 percent in cabbage, 92 percent in lettuce, and 56 percent in spinach. There is little or no iodine in our produce; unless the soils are supplemented with iodine, it is not generally present. Even though kiwi and spinach are reported to be high in iodine, if the soil does not contain it, it cannot be taken into the cells of that plant. Lack of iodine creates problems for human beings; as a result of iodine deficiency in soil, certain disorders appear in the body. Your attention and concentration may be lowered. You may become irritable, depressed, and get tired quickly. Among the other symptoms of iodine deficiency are headaches, short-term memory loss, loss of previous intelligence or problem-solving abilities, lowering of hemoglobin levels in the blood, frequent chills, and, in women, menstrual cycle disorders. In most cases, problematic signs appear little by little, imperceptibly, and gradually. Iodine deficiency is called a "hidden hunger." In children, iodine deficiency provokes hyperactivity, heightened excitability, and mental development challenges. It is not difficult to understand why we have so many thyroid problems in America. Nonbiological chemical iodized salts are often created in a laboratory like a drug and are not used by the body like a true iodine source. That is why I favor sea vegetables like nori, kelp, wakame, kombu, or dulse as a means to absorb iodine and B_{12}. Grind these in the spice grinder to sprinkle like salt, or add them to your green smoothies for added nutrient value. Calcium and iron accumulate at much higher levels in seaweed than in land plants. An eight-gram portion of dried kombu has more calcium than a cup (200 ml) of milk, and dulse contains more iron than sirloin steak. Seaweed alginates and carrageenans are sometimes used to give processed foods like sausages or croissants more flavor and texture. Not that this makes processed foods more acceptable in the daily diet. Most sea vegetables contain amino acids, plus vitamins A, C, and E, and they are one of the few vegetable sources of vitamin B_{12}. That is why I feel these are essential in the raw diet plan. While seaweed is used frequently for healing in traditional Chinese medicine, it unfortunately remains a mystery to industrialized medicine. Research has proven that kombu and wakame have polysaccharides called fucoidans that exhibit anticancer activity. The fiber in sea vegetables has been shown to be beneficial for the digestive system as an anti-inflammatory as well as promoting lipid metabolism. If you do not care for the taste or texture of sea vegetables, learn how to add them to certain foods so you hide the texture or flavor. When our children were young, I would add chopped nori to their vegetable soup.

Author and whole food activist Paul Stitt reports that we lose 90 percent of the mineral content of our food from "garden to gullet." When we cook our produce we further eliminate enzymes and minerals. In 2002, he wrote in the *Journal of the American Medical Association*: "Most people do not consume an optimal amount of all vitamins and minerals by diet alone." This is due to overcooking and consuming overprocessed foods.

MY NINE FAVORITE POWER-PACKED VEGETABLES

Mix them up, but eat at least three from each category weekly!

1. *Beets:* A blood cleanser high in iron, folate, manganese, potassium, and dietary fiber, as well as vitamin C, tryptophan, copper, and phosphorus. Beet greens also contain high amounts of nutrients, including the carotenoids lutein and zeaxanthin.

2. *Kale, broccoli, cabbage, turnips, and Brussels sprouts:* Members of the Brassica family vegetables, which contain phytochemicals that combat cancer, have anti-inflammatory properties, and improve immune function. The nutrients include potassium, vitamins C and K, calcium, folic acid, and iron. Holocaust survivors liberated from concentration camps were health-

ier than most doctors expected because they subsisted on a diet of turnips. Juiced turnips are reputed to clear mucus and the symptoms of asthma.

3. *Red bell peppers:* Contain vitamins A and C; provide protection against rheumatoid arthritis. Vitamin C is essential for the repair and maintenance of cartilage and bones. It is crucial in the formation of collagen, an important protein used to make tendons, cartilage, and ligaments. Vitamin A promotes healthy bone development. Red peppers are also rich in vitamin E and beta-cryptoxanthin, two antioxidants that absorb free radicals (which cause inflammation) while increasing joint flexibility.

4. *Carrots and sweet potatoes:* A cup (200 ml) of raw carrots contains 34,500 IU of vitamin A, the richest vegetable source of pro–vitamin A carotenes. These have been shown to protect vision and reduce the risk of heart disease and certain types of cancers. Both carrots and sweet potatoes are also a very good source of vitamins C and K, fiber, potassium, and B-complex vitamins, manganese, molybdenum, phosphorus, magnesium, and folate.

5. *Spinach (and other dark leafy greens):* Contains more than thirty-five essential vitamins and minerals, including a dozen flavonoids. A cup (200 ml) provides the body with three times the daily value of vitamin A and over 1,000 percent of the recommended daily value of vitamin K.

6. *Garlic and onions:* Should regularly be included in our diets. Garlic contains antioxidants and helps boost immunity. Onion has been shown to have similar positive affects. Both can help fight infection.

7. *Cauliflower:* A good source of protein, thiamine, riboflavin, niacin, magnesium, and phosphorus, plus fiber, vitamins C, K, B_6, folate, pantothenic acid, and manganese.

8. *Edamame, green peas, and beans:* Have more protein than most other vegetables and also contain complex carbohydrates, folate, fiber, calcium, iron, magnesium, and potassium. A cup (200 ml) of lightly steamed, organic soybeans can supply the body with an excellent amount of molybdenum and tryptophan, a substantial amount of manganese and protein, and a good amount of more than ten other essential nutrients, including omega-3 fatty acids, fiber, and potassium. One cup (200 ml) of beans provides more than 50 percent of the required daily value for protein. These must be organic because of the use of hexane, a neurotoxin, in nonorganic processing. Cornucopia, an independent research agency, reports the following:

"Widespread use of hexane is used in soy processing. Hexane is strictly prohibited in organic food processing, but is used to make 'natural' soy foods and even some that are 'made with organic ingredients' . . . Hexane is a neurotoxic petrochemical solvent that is listed as a hazardous air pollutant with the Environmental Protection Agency (EPA)."

9. *Tomatoes:* While really a fruit, tomatoes are very high in antioxidants and lycopene, which are effective in the treatment of prostate cancer and heart disease. Research at Harvard revealed that men who ate tomato-based foods daily had a 35 percent lower risk of developing prostate cancer, and the benefits were more pronounced among those with advanced stages of prostate cancer. In an unrelated study, men taking fifty milligrams (mg) of lycopene daily had significantly lower prostate-specific antigen (PSA) levels, a key marker for prostate cancer. The risk of developing aggressive prostate cancer decreased with increasing lycopene levels.

An article in the journal *Nutrition,* citing animal studies, reported that lycopene, taken at similar doses, was more effective than statin drugs in treating heart disease related to LDL and HDL cholesterol levels. Statin drugs constitute two of the top three best-selling drugs in the United States. You might avoid raw tomatoes if you have a hiatal hernia or gastroesophageal reflux disease (GERD).

Organic tomatoes have almost 57 percent higher levels of lycopene than nonorganic and nearly double the amount of antioxidants. It is important to note that higher levels of lycopene are present in cooked tomatoes: tomato paste has nearly 42.2 milligrams (mg)/100 grams (g) where raw tomatoes contain only 3mg/100g. For that reason, I suggest organic, sugar-free ketchup (those made with agave nectar are fine) on my raw healing diet.

CHAPTER 4

Emotional Food Addiction

*It is much more important to know what sort of a patient
has a disease than what sort of a disease a patient has.*

—WILLIAM OSIER

One of the most dangerous and difficult of all addictions is the addiction to unhealthy foods, since many of our senses are involved in what we eat. It isn't just our taste buds that figure in the process of eating. Taste buds can detect only five flavors: sweet, salty, bitter, sour, and savory, which has also been labeled as *umami*. *Umami* is a Japanese word meaning "savory," a deliciousness factor deriving specifically from detection of the natural amino acid glutamic acid, or glutamates common in meats, cheese, broth, stock, and other protein-heavy foods. The action of umami receptors explains why foods treated with monosodium glutamate (MSG) often taste "heartier." The other senses that influence food selection and consumption are sight, or what looks good; smell; and our sense of taste. Our cravings are a reflection of what our body may be lacking, but our sense of what that nutrient actually is may be misinterpreted. A good example of this is chocolate. No one suffers from a chocolate deficiency. What your body may instead be craving is fruit. Your blood sugar may be low, so a message is sent to your brain. If there is a stressed or an emotional component attached to the message, it is often translated from the basic need for carbohydrates to a desire for something sweet and caffeinated. The sweet-tasting taste buds are located on the tip of your tongue. These are designed to seek out fruits, starches, and vegetables that supply us with energy and healthful nutrition. Unless you eat enough of the proper types of beneficial carbohydrates, you will remain hungry and continue to forage for food. This is where emotional eating has its roots in many people. You cannot trust your taste buds if your body pH is too acidic and you are hanging on by a thread above an emotional abyss, ready to kill for a piece of chocolate. Carl Jung's "dark night of the soul" was not about eating chocolate. We must learn to separate balanced nutrition from emotional desires and stimuli, and seek personal or professional counselors to help us understand those vicious wounds that drive our enteric or gut brain and our emotional eating responses. Emotional wounds drive a wedge between our physical needs and our emotional decisions. If you find yourself mindlessly reaching for that chocolate-chip cookie or beer at the end of the day as a reward for surviving yet another twenty-four hours of life, you are truly punishing yourself. This decision embodies what Alcoholics Anonymous calls *stinkin' thinkin'*. You fabricate exotic excuses to enable bad habits that harm or threaten your health and well-being. We purposely neglect to study the effects of any addiction because we may be forced to turn the emotional rock over and look at where it came from or what it is doing to us. We know that we may be stabbing ourselves in the heart with a fork, but we seem powerless to stop because we don't know who we are without the addiction. We "need" our comfort foods. Humans are naturally inclined to crave carbohydrates. But if we turn that statement over to highlight making food bad choices or eating junk food, it translates to: "I've got an internal sabotage program running and I am getting something out of it." The quest then becomes to define what that emotional poltergeist is before it brings on disease or death. Red meat, poultry, and shellfish contain no carbohydrates, and dairy products and eggs contains very little. People who eat a diet rich in animal-based foods are never truly satisfied and become compulsive overeaters. They do not know that sometimes just eating an apple would satisfy their deep cravings much more than eating a pint of ice cream or a fast-food burger. One example of extreme emotional food addiction was a new patient, Bob, who came to my office with a recent diagnosis of colon cancer at the age of 49. The majority of his diet consisted of red meat, and with that he often ate French fries. He proudly called himself the king of the fast-food drive-through. I asked him why he chose to eat this way, and he responded that it was fast and easy, a "no-brainer." He always ordered the supersized portions and got a good deal for his buck. Bob was much too busy with his sales job to bother with the purchase, preparation, or proper consumption of food. "You can't ever argue with cheap, fast, and easy, Doc," he insisted. But there was something else underlying his words. There was an emotional denial. I recognized that Bob did not seem to like himself and found lots of obvious excuses to avoid nurturing many of his other basic needs. When the buck stopped at cancer, his response was, "We all die of something. Mine's probably gonna be cancer. My old man died of a heart attack at fifty-six; I always figured that would be how I would go." Bob's answers were too fast and detached. He had made up his mind that this was it: his death was inevitable, and he was in no mood to change his old habits or take care of himself. When he was seven years old, his parents divorced. Meals at the dinner table disappeared from his life when his mother was forced to go back to work. Bob's exhausted mother would bring him a bag of nearly cold drive-through food for dinner on her way home from the factory. That bag of food was a mother doing her best to keep her child's stomach full. When he told me this story, his eyes filled with tears. He adapted to the divorce, but lost the ability to accept nurturing. He rarely saw his father after that, since Bob's father had remarried and had a new family to connect to. Bob said that he was a stale leftover in his own father's eyes. All his life, that was the perspective Bob had of himself. He was alone most of his life after his father left. Bob shared with me that it was his father who taught him that vegetables were for sissies. Meat was for real men. The unfortunate side effect of this twisted philosophy was that it probably killed both of them. Bob stated that he would rather die than change his dietary habits, and so he did. It seems unfortunate to me when an individual dies without healing emotional wounds from his past, but even more devastating when the wounds could be recognized and healed before death.

Meat can be more addictive that sugar, and if meat is overconsumed, it can be lethal. I find it a sad fact that the more ill a person is, the less likely she is to be able to alter her diet. More than any other food, red meat has the potential to create a deleterious **or harmful** change in the chemistry of the brain. Overconsumption of red meat has been blamed for wars and prison riots. An interesting experiment was conducted in a prison in Sweden. The detainees were all fed a vegetarian diet for three months. At the end of that period, the following facts were gathered: violence was nearly eliminated during that period and aggression was down overall. Unfortunately, the prison went back its old diet after the study was completed.

Protein is synthesized by the liver into blood urea nitrogen. The kidneys must filter out this urea. Excess urea causes enlargement of the kidneys, and this can cause damage to the tubeoles of the kidneys. If you have diabetes or high blood pressure, excessive protein consumption may lead to tissue damage that ultimately destroys the kidneys. Many people do not consume enough water to flush urea out of the body. Another nitrogen-producing aspect of protein breakdown is ammonia. Excess ammonia in the intestines can cause cancer. Excess animal protein also leeches calcium from the bones. While medical doctors are busy pushing 1,200-plus milligrams of calcium on older women, they seem oblivious to the fact that excess animal protein consumption causes severe calcium deficiency. According to *The Vegetarian Handbook,* by Gary Null, Americans, on average, consume about 200 pounds (91 kg) of red meat, 50 pounds (23 kg) of chicken and turkey, 10 pounds (4.5 kg) of assorted fish, 300 eggs, and 250 pounds (114 kg) of dairy products a year. This is four times the amount of protein recommended daily. The USDA data confirms that the average American over a lifetime consumes 21,000 animals. The result can be deadly: cancer of the breast, colon, or prostate; heart, liver, and kidney disease; as well as obesity.

Several years ago, I had the opportunity to meet Howard Lyman, "the Mad Cowboy." He is famous for the lawsuit that followed his interview on television by Oprah Winfrey. Oprah said that she would never eat another hamburger. The cattle industry was furious about that comment. Howard and his wife are vegetarians. He was a rancher, but also a chemist. When he discovered that he had life-threatening cancer, he did some long-overdue research. He discovered that the chemically treated feed and pesticides, antibiotics, sodium nitrate, BHT, and BHA hormones fed to and injected into cattle probably contribute to human cancer. He also theorized that much of what is now called Alzheimer's disease is actually misdiagnosed bovine encephalitis, or mad cow disease. We test the blood of very few cows for this disease before they are slaughtered and sent to the market for human consumption. In Japan, every single meat animal is tested. Even though most Americans are not aware of this fact, cloned beef need not be labeled before being sold to the public. So when I have a sick patient ask me what I have against meat, I never know where to begin with a response.

If you are healthy and would like to eat animal protein sparingly, the impact of that choice is not as threatening as it is for someone who has an active disease process that must be reversed as soon as possible. In a *Washington Post* article titled "Daily Red Meat Raises Chances of Dying Early," dated March 24, 2009, research from the National Cancer Institute indicated that

"The bottom line is, we found an association between red meat and processed meat and an increased risk of mortality." The study was based on evidence from more than 500,000 middle-aged and elderly Americans who consumed about four ounces (113 g) of red meat a day, or the equivalent of a small hamburger. During the ten years they were followed, 30 percent of these people were more likely to die, mostly from heart disease and cancer. This new study not only confirmed previous research that red meat increased the risk of cancer and heart disease but is the first new study that examines the relationship between eating meat and overall risk of death. It is a very detailed study. It concluded that eating red meat increases the chances of dying prematurely, and it's the first large study to examine whether regularly eating beef or pork increases mortality. "The uniqueness of this study is its size and length of follow-up," said Barry M. Popkin, a professor of global nutrition at the University of North Carolina, who wrote an editorial accompanying the study. "This is a slam-dunk to say that, 'Yes, indeed, if people want to be healthy and live longer, consume less red and processed meat.' " There are many reasons that overconsumption of red meat might be unhealthy: cooking or grilling red meat generates cancer-causing compounds; red meat is high in saturated fat, which has been associated with breast and colorectal cancer; and meat is very high in excessive iron, also believed to promote cancer. Also, people who eat red meat are more likely to have high blood pressure and cholesterol, which increases the risk of heart disease. Processed meats may contain carcinogenic compounds. Meat has a very acidic pH, and people who consume meat often eat it with bread or potatoes. This inhibits the body's ability to digest properly. This is considered bad food combining. In addition to this problem, individuals who consume excessive meat often neglect to eat a nutritious amount of fruits and vegetables.

Healthy children do not naturally start their lives craving highly processed, addictive foods, but are more interested in fruits. Eating processed breads, sweets, and hamburgers is a learned behavior. In some cases, this behavior can begin in the womb. Newborns are fed mother's breast milk, which is ideal, but a number of studies indicate that most American breast milk is contaminated with hazardous toxins. Processed formulas or powders are mainly sweetened toxic substances with no enzymes whatsoever; hydrogen peroxide tests have proven that even the best created formulas have no enzymes to aid in the digestive processes. (I suggest real organic goat's milk with liquid vitamins added.) After early infancy, babies are fed processed baby foods in a jar that are often enhanced with sweeteners. Addictive foods only get worse from there. Look at some of the ingredients in processed foods. If you cannot pronounce the names of the chemical ingredients, your body probably doesn't know what to do with them. Eating these chemicals might be thought of as slowly embalming yourself. From time to time, we have people who do not know us well "gift" us with nonorganic, processed sweets. We simply bless the good thoughts and intentions of the giver and compost or recycle the products. I tell patients who have junk in their pantry to get rid of it as soon as possible in whatever way besides eating it that can make them feel less guilty. Making healthier choices immediately allows your body to heal faster.

One major food manufacturing company is owned by a major tobacco company. Company officials have learned how to get people addicted to their products. They transferred the same formulas for addiction from tobacco to foods, but instead of using nicotine, they used refined fats, sugars, and wheat flour. These foods are physiologically addictive, and once addicted, you feel repeatedly drawn to consume them. Switching away from these addictive foods may seem difficult in the beginning. Your mind will try to convince you that a raw diet is threatening, and this puts your coping mechanisms on alert to shy away from raw foods. That is where you need support from others, or the knowledge that you have been manipulated into ill health may make you angry enough to persevere. Remember that you won't get that drugged or medicated feeling that you get from toxic, processed foods. Your body will have the opportunity, perhaps for the first time in your life, to purge itself of the bad foods that have adhered as plaque to your colon. Self-medicating with food also spikes emotional resistance. There is a definite shock to the system, similar to no longer taking a drug that you have used your entire life; you will have a withdrawal symptoms, so prepare yourself to deal with it in a rational way.

EMOTIONAL EATING AND THE THREE GUNAS

Yogis believe that all food affects the body and the mind. They feel that the fear of death is able to permeate every cell of an animal's body before and when it is slaughtered. Eating the flesh of dead animals violates the first principle of yamas, or yogic ethics, as laid down in the Yoga Sutras, or laws, by Patanjali. That is the law of nonviolence, or *ahimsa*.

The traditional yogic diet is considered to be a lacto-vegetarian eating regimen that avoids eggs as well as all animal flesh. They consider that proteins that can be obtained from nuts, dairy products, and legumes are generally of a higher quality than those from meat. Food is classified using the three Gunas: the Sattva, the Raja, and the Tamas.

Sattvic foods are primarily what they call sweet, fresh, and agreeable. These include leafy green vegetables and other vegetables, fruits, nuts, seeds, whole grains, and honey, plus pure water and raw milk as beverages. The emotions that accompany a consumption of this diet are life affirming, more open, compassionate, and positive. This is the diet that is most favorable for spiritual growth and brings peace to life.

Rajasic foods create restlessness in the mind and are avoided by most yoga practitioners. These include spicy and stimulating foods, like meat, fish, all processed foods, chocolate, garlic, onions, eggs, coffee, and tea. Eating too fast or with a disturbed or stressed mind is also considered rajasic. The emotions that accompany raja are obsession, including feeling attached and overly passionate about things, anxiety, and panic.

Tamasic food is thought to be poisonous. It creates a dullness of the mind and obscures the thinking. It involves overconsuming the wrong kinds of foods that are dead, stale, and overripe. This diet includes alcohol, processed foods and meats, and few or no fresh foods. Mental and emotional inertia, feeling stuck and dark inside, rage, ignorance, and faulty actions are associated with this diet.

Yogis believe that the nature of food can change by cooking it. Cooking is the most obvious way to change the nature of food. Grains become sattvic after cooking. Honey becomes tamasic or poisonous when cooked. The nature of food also changes by combining it with other foods and spices, or if it is stored for protracted periods. Fruits shouldn't be eaten when they are overripe because they rot and become tamasic.

How to eat and when to eat are also important considerations for yogis. A person should not eat too late at night. There should be a gap of at least two to four hours between the last meal of the day and sleep. Food should always be freshly prepared and eaten with attention, respect, and gratitude. Leftovers are never consumed. Food should be delicious, so as to be appreciated. The attitude of the person preparing the food is important as well, as the mood of the cook permeates the food. I heard that it was the practice of Yogananda to always pick the happiest or most peaceful person in the crowd to prepare food for the next meal. Most yogis still prefer their meals prepared at home to meals prepared in a restaurant to ensure that the emotional status and spirituality of the chef are of high quality and the chef exudes happiness.

EAT A HIGH-QUALITY FRESH DIET

On this raw healing diet, you eat only raw fruits and vegetables, nuts, grains, and seeds. I will explain later what is important to eat every day for proper pH and to meet your body's optimum need for vital nutrients. You will not miss a single nutrient in this diet, and you will achieve optimum wellness.

Recently, a very competent nutritionist brought a gentle and kind patient, Joan, in for a consultation. Joan had been clinically tested with blood, saliva, and urine and found that she could not tolerate the limited range of processed foods that she had been eating most of her life. Her diet was essentially gluten-based, and my philosophy is that if a person eliminates gluten grains from her diet, she may be better able to tolerate other blacklisted food items. This sensitive patient was truly an emotional eater who seemed to have a great deal of adrenal activity related to her eating habits: she ate like a rushed freshman in a high school cafeteria, wolfing down a hasty bag of food. I call this "fight-or-flight feeding." Joan said that she often woke up with the message, "I have to eat something, and I have to eat it now!" So she would grab a peanut butter sandwich or a candy bar for breakfast. Not only was this quick and convenient, but it represented comfort food for her, a reminder of the better days from her childhood. But she ate foodless foods with emotional petulance, cramming big bites into her mouth and swallowing it without chewing. Emotional habits and wounds can be paralyzing, and developing new patterns may seem overwhelming. While it is vital to recognize why negative emotional eating habits persist, it is equally imperative to use this dysfunctional information to create a new functional path for positive eating. When eating becomes a mechanism to quiet the emotional dragon inside, as it was in Joan's case, it is necessary to nurture and understand what food really represents to this individual. There are lots of people who act like Joan, and not just when it comes to eating.

Several years ago, I treated a patient who so loathed bowel movements that she would put them off for several days, fretting and making herself sick with urgency. When she finally succumbed, she had a difficult time going, she felt trapped between the desire to escape the dreaded bathroom and the need to stay to adequately empty her bowels. Why are people caught in these strange emotional webs of their own creation? I've come to the conclusion that the answer lies in their past, and recognized or unconscious stressors in their current life keep them locked in a particular dysfunctional pattern.

There is a stress hormone called gherlin that actually mimics hunger and makes a person feel as if he is hungry or that he must eat something—anything—as soon as possible. If you have too much stress in your life, you may find yourself eating more just to appease the urgent cry of this particular hormone. When our bodies send out hunger signals, levels of ghrelin—that appetite-stimulating hormone—increase. According to a recent study, funded in part by the National Institutes of Health, ghrelin's main function may not be letting you know it's time for a snack as much as it is used to fight stress. Using mice, researchers experimented with ghrelin levels by restricting calories and giving injections of the hormone that, over time, made the mice numb to ghrelin's appetite-stimulating effects. These mice ultimately became depressed and suicidal. When our bodies send out hunger signals or signals of stress, ghrelin levels rise. We are prompted to eat because the mixed signal to do so is present and becomes almost a fight-or-flight stimulus. We must recognize our response to stress and find a way to understand the biochemical messages that dictate our eating habits.

Sleeping patterns also are related to stress and weight retention. Recent research indicates that sleeping 7 $1/2$ hours a night helps calm stress that promotes the tendency to be overweight. If you have trouble getting to sleep, you are probably locked in either a stress-related cortisol elevation cycle or you're beginning to feel the effects of an autoimmune disease process. While these two are related, it is important to investigate how to better manage your daily stress, and how to change emotionally based dietary choices, as ways to get a better night's sleep.

In *Coyote Medicine,* Lewis Mehl-Madrona shared a medicine man's philosophy: "Before a person can be healed, he or she must answer three simple questions: 'Who are you?' 'Where did you come from?' and 'Why are you here?'" It was believed that anyone who could answer these questions clearly would get well. If you regularly reach for "comfort foods," such as meat or white, denatured foods, you might want to explore the possibility that you are trying to find something outside yourself to feel whole. The addictive relationship with food takes us outside of our emotional self and may even provide a mood alteration for a short time. Shame or guilt often accompany this pattern. You may see yourself as a victim of past circumstances and bound to bad habits that ultimately take control of you. Part of this problem may be a positive or negative emotional link to your past. Maybe you remember the milk and cookies that your adoring grandmother set out for you after school, and after a rough day at work you feel you owe yourself a latte and a piece of cheesecake. This is a positive memory, but with a negative outcome. Your younger self seized emotional control and is not making very wise, healing choices about food. Many times food is used as a ritual or communion with loved ones, and you are missing the positive ritual of that experience. What you might benefit from is considering that your adult self is capable of making conscious choices to heal and nurture the body, mind, spirit, and emotions. The answer to the "Who are you?" question above then becomes, "I am an adult who needs to feel loved or adored by another confirming human being." The answer to "Where did you come from?" might be: "I came from a broken family where my grandmother was the one person who cared enough to be there for me, to listen to me, and to support me." And the answer to "Why are you here?" then becomes: "I recognize that I am not strong enough to cope with this issue on my own. I need help and support to overcome my addiction to foods that are feeding my disease. Please help me, I need help. I don't have the emotional tools to heal this addiction, and I feel ashamed of my health issues because I have neglected to take care of myself." In Debbie Ford's book, titled *The Dark Side of the Light Chasers,* she asks this question: "Who's driving your emotional bus?" In the case above, it would probably be a nine-year-old. What nine-year-old child wouldn't choose cookies and candy over vegetables and fruit? You need to put the adult in charge. For that to happen, you need to experience emotional healing.

After any dietary change, there is generally an emotional response. I always tell patients that they may feel the emotional effects of frustration or grieving after they leave behind foods they have been addicted to emotionally for one reason or another. While some may feel sad and depressed for a short period, others become agitated and annoyed, frustrated and angry. Giving up sugar and white foods, in particular, causes emotional storms because these foods are related to yeasty beasties in the body that demand to be fed. Two days after a dietary change, one aggravated patient called to say that she hated the "gloppy green smoothie" that I suggested she eat for breakfast and hated, hated, hated all greens and fruits. She then proceeded to throw a whining tantrum on the telephone. I waited patiently, saying nothing, until she said to me in a five-year-old voice, "This is all your fault." I could nearly see her little finger pointing at me. I asked her how old she felt just now. And I asked her when she last felt this way. She reported that it was when her father had abandoned the family and her mother had to return to work. She ate cereal, cookies, and crackers from a box for two meals a day. She suddenly realized that she had been feeding the wound of her five-year-old self. It was time to heal the wound of the past and no longer allow her father's abandonment to ruin the rest of her life. She invested energy in the three healing questions, and we arrived at three powerful affirmations together. I will share them with you. Then I suggest that you formulate your own positive, present-tense affirmations to help you overcome food addictions and find your path to nurturing with raw, enzyme-rich, healing foods.

1. **"Who are you?"** Suggested comprehensive affirmation: "I am a wise, empowered woman who nurtures herself daily with raw vegetables and fruit. I feel the effects of an enzyme-rich, healing diet, and my body, mind, spirit, and emotions are balanced and in harmony with healing. I deserve to feel healthy, and I take responsibility to provide myself with and accept healing foods."

   - "But this is too hard." This translates into "I am not motivated enough to change my old patterns." Affirm: "I embrace change and am excited about learning new ways to nurture myself. As I learn how to prepare new foods, I am inspired by the new flavors that feed my soul and nurture my mind and body."

   - "This is expensive." This translates into a lack of understanding. Affirm: "I know that I am worthy of the cost of organic produce because it creates the sense of health and well-being in my body that I deserve.

   - "I don't have the tools." The underlying sentiment is related to self-sabotage and self-limiting behavior from the past. Affirm: "I know that I have all that I need to support my new healing lifestyle. This is more than a diet; this is a move to health and healing."

2. **"Where did you come from?"** Suggested comprehensive affirmation: "I recognize that in the past I used food for emotional support and comfort. I now use food as fuel and for healing. I love fresh vegetables and fruits, and I feel the difference in my own empowerment to make wise food choices."

   - "I need my old food habits as a connection to my ethnic family." This translates into "I am not worthy of my own personal identity and health." Affirm: "I came from a place where poor food choices created diseases in my family. I recognize that I can convert any recipe into a healthy ethnic treasure to share with my loved ones."

- "If I change my old diet, what will I eat?" This translates into a lack of desire to change old, destructive habits. This also translates into investing in the diseases that may plague your natal family. Affirm: "I honor my mind by allowing it the potential to research and develop a new plan for eating that is enticing and exciting. I look forward to planning and preparing meals, rather than continuing the sedentary lifestyle of my past."

3. **"Why are you here?"** Suggested comprehensive affirmation: "I have awakened to a new lifestyle that nurtures my body, mind, spirit, and emotions. I heal now with fresh, raw vegetables and fruit. It is time. Enough is enough."

   - "I can change little things and still eat my chocolate, bagels, and red meat." This translates into delusional thinking. The child self is taking control, using addictive thinking to hold onto the past. Affirm: "I am more than ready to change. I give myself the gift of healing and compassion. I deserve love from myself to nurture and support my healing process. I am enough."

   - "Diabetes isn't so bad. There are worse things that could happen." This translates into denial. Diabetes and the synthetic drugs used now to treat it can lead to kidney failure. Affirm: "I see the bigger picture in a long, healthy, disease-free life. I am responsible for the quality of my life. I affirm life with good healthy eating habits. I enjoy fresh fruits and vegetables."

Recently, I received a call from a woman who wanted to know if I treated individuals with diabetes. I explained that it is my goal to help patients heal their diabetes by making better nutritional choices. I was shocked at her reply: "I don't want you to help me to heal my diabetes. I just want you to help me to treat it." If you find yourself paralyzed in what might be considered unhealthy eating habits, please consider drug-free counseling or hypnosis to get beyond your stress and the blocks that get in the way of your health and wellness. I might also recommend John Bradshaw's books or CDs about ego state therapy, also known as healing your inner child.

When I work in my practice with people who have suffered emotional or traumatic experiences, I often think of the ancient shamanic awareness of something called "soul loss." When we experience a great loss or emotional injury, tragedy, or injustice, we feel that loss in our heart or in our gut. Many times I have listened as patients tell me about a hole in their heart after a loved

AN EMOTIONAL RAW FOODS STORY

—KM, WISCONSIN

I made some significant changes in my life, and my eating habits were among those changes. In 2001 I began the journey of changes. I was eating poorly, I traveled a lot for business, and I ate the Standard American Diet, not knowing any better. I thought I felt good and that my health was generally fine. I had frequent sinus infections, headaches, trouble breathing, and achy joints. I weighed approximately 210 pounds (95 kg). Emotionally, I was a wreck; I cried frequently, I had no passion for life, and I felt no joy. I was irritable and tired. I was told that I needed to make changes or I would not be here to make changes, and I still fought the changes. Dr. Mitchell told me that I should try a raw food diet and soon I would be able to eat the foods that I wanted. I remember asking how long it would be before I could eat what I wanted, picturing a blueberry pie and a cookie in my head.

I took my first raw food class with Dr. Mitchell and began to change my diet. I eliminated what I could easily and introduced more raw foods into my diet. I began eating more salads and started walking three to five days a week for thirty minutes on my lunch hour. Time factors were an issue; I had to decide what I could change easily without taking more time to prepare. Some changes came when I had saved to buy a dehydrator or food processor. I still ate some cooked foods, but I found that if I stayed away from something for three to four weeks and tried it again, I did not enjoy it and it made me feel sluggish or tired. Along the way, I also shifted to eating organic as much as possible. I lost eighty pounds (36 kg) over three to four years with this change in my eating habits and exercise, and I have maintained my weight within five pounds (2 kg) for four years now.

I feel healthier and stronger since I have made the changes. I no longer get headaches or have trouble breathing. Emotionally, I feel joy; I am no longer depressed. I became stronger emotionally and changed careers. Changing my diet and working with art therapy created a new and healthy balance emotionally. My focus is to work on the mental, physical, emotional, and spiritual balance, since they are all connected. If you race ahead and work on only one piece, something will strain to catch up or pull the other pieces out of balance. I currently eat 75 to 80 percent raw. With the right tools, the raw food preparation takes the same or less time than cooked foods. Soups in the blender are much quicker. The cooked foods I eat are soups or vegetable dishes when the weather outside is cold or damp.

When I look back at what my health was like before, I realize that I really was not healthy, but I didn't know any better. My energy level has increased significantly; people comment frequently on how healthy and happy I look. I am healthy and confident. "I want what you have" is what I hear several times a month. Occasionally, I still get old cravings as I detoxify the old layers of toxins. Most of the time I can let them go, but if I eat something that is not feeding me, I can feel it emotionally and physically within hours. The cleaner my system, the healthier I am and the more aware I am that my body lets me know how what I eat affects it. Now I can eat the foods that I want, but I no longer want cookies or a blueberry pie—I want the fresh, healthy, raw foods that make me feel like I am truly alive."

one has died, or about a visceral pain gnawing at their insides. Unfortunately, without strong emotional support, people try to fill that hole or stop the gnawing at the gut with sugar-based foods or alcohol. These quickly become addictive because the acids offer a quick fix for emotional pain. Emotional potholes are part of the road of life and must be repaired from the inside out. All that you gain from throwing addictive foods into the mix is weight and disease. I share compassionately with my patients the truth that they do not have to suffer for the rest of their lives for a negative emotional event that occurred in their past. Henry David Thoreau said, "Most men lead lives of quiet desperation and go to the grave with the song still in them." I believe that the majority of us live lives of quiet desperation, but I also believe that we have a choice to alter or change that. You choose a life script, as Eric Berne called it, based on living out an emotionally disabled life as a form of chronic suicide. You may play the role of the victim according to the life script you have chosen. I feel that we each have the innate power to understand that we no longer need to accept the role of victim. Life continues, and part of that continuation is a conscious choice that we make when we get out of bed every morning. On some level, we can choose happiness or we can choose to be unhappy, to be a victim or to be someone who consciously chooses to be otherwise. I also share with my patients that healthy nutrition in organic fruits and vegetables are great allies for emotional healing. The victim in you may choose addictive foods because you feel that you can't empower a healthy consciousness. The victim in you may feel and appear to be very young and powerless. You must decide to put your adult self in charge of making good food choices. To put this in perspective, consider that, given a choice, children generally choose foods with a lot of sugar. You may function at work or at home as an adult, making important decisions mentally and financially, but emotionally the injured child inside you may be driving you to distraction. Your five- or seven-year-old self may guide you consciously or unconsciously to the bakery aisle, but the adult self must redirect that younger you toward the fresh produce. I always ask patients with food disorders who is in charge of making up the shopping list. While they're confused at first, about my intention in asking, they soon realize that they have the power, as adults, to choose good nutrition. Feeding emotional wounds ultimately makes us feel more vulnerable than ever. If you have this book in your hands, you are taking a large step toward personal empowerment and healing.

We must also recognize the connection between the mind and food on a deeper level. The enteric brain of the digestive system, or the "gut brain," as it has been called, records and remembers positive and negative emotions. Since its nerve cells are affected by the same protein messengers as the brain itself, the brain and the gut can upset each other. Dr. Michael Gershon, professor of cellular biology at Columbia Presbyterian Medical Center in New York, has studied the system of cells and major neurotransmitters of serotonin, dopamine, glutamate, and norepinephrine found lining the digestive organs. He notes that 95 percent of the body's serotonin, the antidepressive, happiness neurotransmitter, is found in the enteric brain. Gershon said, "The enteric brain plays a major role in human happiness and misery." Years or months of stress, repressed emotions, and trauma can put the enteric brain into a state of chronic digestive and emotional chaos. This creates a disaster for health and healing and can even upset immune regulation and promote disease processes. Unfortunately, these effects are unconscious: Individuals may suffer for many years and yet be unaware that they are barely surviving and are in a state of deep depression.

The wife of a sixty-five-year-old man made an appointment with me for physical and emotional assistance regarding their thirty-two-year-old daughter's death several years earlier. Ted was extremely withdrawn and shared only that he felt as if he had a hole in his heart ever since his daughter had died. He was suffering from CHF, congestive heart failure. He was so steeped in anguish and was so remote that he was not responding to the questions that I asked him. I discovered from his wife that Ted had a desire to eat only cinnamon rolls and prepackaged bakery sweets. His daughter loved cinnamon buns, his wife explained, and it was their last meal together. Her distraught comment to me was, "He has to eat something." I asked them both if that is all that they would feed their daughter if she was still alive. "Of course not" was the response. I took the next emotional step with them and suggested that true healing only occurs when a person wants to get well. I would never try to rush or drastically limit a person's grieving process, but Ted was punishing himself for something he had no control over. Ted couldn't protect his daughter from her death. I told him that his wife and daughter would not want him to suffer this way. I mentioned to Ted that he may not be honoring his daughter's life nor helping his wife with her stress by not taking care of himself or trying to live, rather than die. Of course, he had not thought in these terms before, since the emotional pain and his poor diet limited his mental processes and perspective. They agreed to try a raw diet for three months. He agreed to let go of his daily focus on suffering and guilt over his daughter's death. We created an affirmation for Ted to repeat three times a day: "My heart is healing every day with happiness and fresh vegetables and fruit. I live the life my daughter would want for me, and I let myself smile and be happy." As they left, Ted's wife had my 4-3-2-1 Raw Diet guidelines tucked into her purse. She said, "I sure hope this diet works. Nothing else has." I responded that it works, but you have to change old, bad habits to make it work. "I'm going home to throw out the rolls," she claimed. I hope she did.

It is okay to ask for and seek professional help. If professional help isn't available or an option for you, books or CDs can sometimes be a great ally in healing. I have created two CDs for such purposes: one is titled *Heal Now,* for healing the past, and the other is called *Reboot Your Brain,* to deal with the ravages of stress. Keeping a journal also helps you understand how food affects your emotional and physical body; note how you feel after eating certain foods. Love yourself enough to learn how to nurture wellness in your own body and mind. Ask yourself what you really want when you think in terms of emotionally charged foods. Then be aware of how emotion acts and feels in your body, as well as how and where unexpressed emotions are stored. When I took my first psychology course as a sophomore at the University of Iowa, emotions were considered virtually impossible to define, except in terms of conflicting theories. I have since learned that when a person's emotions remain an abstraction to them, they seem unreal and cannot be identified or healed. We must understand what we are feeling and express it in a safe way in a space that we feel is safe.

CHAPTER 5

Can Food Cause Cancer?

"Could cancer lose its grip on modern societies if they turned to a balanced vegetarian diet? The answer is 'yes,' according to two major reports, one by the World Cancer Research Fund and the other by the Committee on the Medical Aspects of Food and Nutrition Policy in the United Kingdom. The reports conclude that a diet rich in plant foods and the maintenance of a healthy body weight could annually prevent four million cases of cancer worldwide."

—ANDREAS MORITZ, *NATURAL NEWS*,
MARCH 30, 2009.

Food must be the most conscious choice that you make, for what you eat sustains your life. Food must also be eaten consciously. If you drive through a fast-food establishment and snag a bag of food, your stomach does not have time to create the digestive environment and secrete the gastric juices necessary for good digestion. If you eat while driving, you are probably gulping rather than chewing forty times to mix amalyse-rich saliva with food to ensure the first stage of digestion. Food plummets down the esophagus to land in the first part of your stomach, where it is supposed to be greeted by and mingled with those digestive enzymes and fluids. Instead of being digested, foods consumed in a manic haste tends to mold. The stomach swells, and incompletely chewed, molding food particles are moved to the second part of the stomach in preparation to be evacuated from the pylorus into the small intestine. Year after year, if your body is assaulted or "punched" with unchewed, partially digested, processed, enzyme-less foods, gastroesophageal reflux disease

51

(GERD) or pyloric insufficiency may develop. Who really teaches us how to eat or what to eat? Is it that same anonymous group of individuals who teach us the other crucial aspects of life? Just last week, I had a cancer patient sincerely share her thoughts: "In school we learn algebra. I have never used it once since. Why didn't I have a single class in school teach me about healthy eating? Why are we led to believe that food has absolutely nothing to do with the creation of disease? In spite of the cancer industry's persistent denial, diseases like cancer generally do not fall out of the sky and land on a person. I know better now how to prevent cancer from ever coming back by making better food choices."

In natural medicine, we consider the disease of cancer to be a toxic process. We clean our houses and we clean our cars, but we are never taught to clean the inside our own bodies. The natural cleansing process of detoxification is ensured if you eat plenty of fiber and enzyme-rich raw vegetables and fruit.

About a year ago, I gained a valuable insight into the American mindset about cancer. While at a chain store that specialized in organic foods, I was asked by the twenty-something-year-old clerk why we wasted our money on organic foods. At first I was a bit shocked by the employee's question, considering where she was working. I related to her how my grandmother, my mother, and my aunt had all died from cancer, and that my cousin now suffered from lung cancer, even though she had never smoked. I told her that my years of research indicated that there was a link between pesticides and breast cancer, and that it is estimated that one in eight women now may develop breast cancer. I also told her that organic, chemical-free vegetables just tasted better, especially carrots and bananas. I told her that monkeys who generally eat the skins of bananas will not touch a banana that is not organic. If they're starving, they will peel the nonorganic banana first and discard the peeling. The clerk gave me an apathetic look and replied, "Look, everyone has to take their turn with cancer." I told her that I was sorry she felt that was the case. Somewhere along the way she had gotten the impression that no matter what we do, we will have to accept cancer as a fact of life. This young clerk was quite invested in her belief that there is no correlation between the food or pesticides that we eat and cancer. Her mother had just lost all her hair, following rounds of chemotherapy. She felt doomed. It is no wonder that Americans feel confused about what to eat to prevent cancer. The American Cancer Society information online link states that:

The term *organic* is popularly used to designate plant foods grown without pesticides and genetic modifications. At this time, no research exists to demonstrate whether such foods are more effective in reducing cancer risk than are similar foods produced by other farming methods. Pesticides and herbicides can be toxic when used improperly in industrial, agricultural, or other occupational settings. Although vegetables and fruits sometimes contain low levels of these chemicals, overwhelming scientific evidence supports the overall health benefits and cancer-protective effects of eating vegetables and fruits. At present there is no evidence that residues of pesticides and herbicides at the low doses found in foods increase the risk of cancer, but fruits and vegetables should be washed thoroughly before eating.

However, in spite of the desire to prove otherwise, researchers continue to find higher concentrations of pesticide levels in the blood serum of breast cancer patients than in controls. In her book, *Pesticides and Breast Cancer: A Wake Up Call,* Dr. Meriel Watts states:

Breast cancer incidence rose 30 to 40 percent from the 1970s to the 1990s. It has been estimated that more than 80 percent of breast cancer cases are associated with environmental factors that include exposure to contaminants, lifestyle, and diet. There is considerable international concern that some of the 70,000 synthetic chemicals in our environment today may be directly linked to a large percentage of breast cancer cases. It has been observed that breast cancer incidence in Western countries has paralleled the proliferation of synthetic chemicals since World War II, and that as developing countries take up industrial agricultural practices, their breast cancer rates escalate similarly.

Dr. Watts's book identifies ninety-eight pesticides, one adjuvant, and two contaminants that may be implicated in the global breast cancer epidemic. She goes on to explain the conundrum of proof: "Scientifically it is impossible to prove that a particular pesticide does or does not cause breast cancer. It never will be proven. Regrettably this does not mean that the pesticides aren't causing breast cancer. It is vital that the government develop a specific breast cancer strategy which recognizes the role of synthetic chemicals in breast cancer, and adopt a precautionary approach to chemicals for which there is evidence of a link with breast cancer, ensuring their replacement with safer alternatives."

I have had the opportunity in the past year to meet many individuals who feel that they have saved their lives from cancer by adopting a raw foods diet. Here is one account from John, an instructor at Northern Illinois University:

In May 2001, I was diagnosed with esophageal cancer. After chemotherapy and radiation, I'd had enough, and though doctors told me that having my esophagus removed was my best chance of a cure, I refused surgery. I knew I had to do something else. I wanted to do the most healing thing for my body. I elected to do a one-month juice and herb fast (cleanse). After finishing that, my tumor turned pink instead of lacerated, but it still was the same size. So I elected to begin a raw food diet: raw, organic fruits, vegetables, nuts, and seeds. That's it. But what I discovered was a whole new way of eating. I attended seminars, read books full of recipes, and discovered that raw food is far more than salads and apples. With books like Nomi Shannon's *Raw Gourmet,* and Juliano Brotman's *Raw: The Uncook Book,* I found that all my meals tasted wonderful and I no longer missed cooked food. After six months, my doctor could not believe the results of my biopsy and endoscopic ultrasound. I was cancer-free and my tumor had reduced itself to only some radiation scar tissue. It's been a year and a half now and I feel better than I have in my entire life. Ironically, cancer was a blessing.

I have conducted a great deal of personal research on the raw foods diet and have found that there is much evidence to support such a healing diet. In 1930, researchers in Lausanne, Switzerland, under the direction of Dr. Paul Kouchakoff, discovered a reaction to cooked foods that they labeled *pathological leukocytosis.* They tested many different types of foods and found that cooked, processed, or refined food immediately caused a rise in the number of white blood cells, or leukocytes. Such a negative reaction in the blood is generally found when the body has been invaded by a dangerous pathogen or suffered a trauma. The researchers were aware of digestive leukocytosis, but the interesting aspect of their research was that this phenomenon did not occur with the ingestion of raw foods. They concluded that the body views cooked and altered foods as a potential pathogen that can harm the blood.

Alan Green, M.D., turned his attention to organic foods when his wife was diagnosed with breast cancer. He tells this story about a study of suburban children living outside of Seattle, conducted by the Department of Environmental Health, University of Washington, and published in 2002 in the newsletter of the *National Institute of Environmental Health Sciences:*

We've known from earlier studies that pesticides and toxic chemicals aren't just in the environment, but get into our developing children's bodies. Some kids have high levels and others quite low. What's different between these kids? Is there anything simple and practical that parents can do to lower their own children's risks? In this study children were divided into two groups: those who ate mostly conventional foods and those who ate mostly organic foods. All urine for twenty-four hours was collected from each child. Children who ate conventional diets had mean pesticide concentrations in their urine nine times higher than the children who ate organic! Their levels indicated that they had exceeded safe exposure levels set by the EPA and were at increased risk to their health. By contrast, those children who ate organic foods were well within the EPA levels deemed to cause negligible risk. Feeding children organic foods is something simple and practical parents can do right now to protect their children and help them build healthy bodies.

Leukocytosis challenges the energy of the body to such a degree that it can make a person feel sleepy or delay the healing process. Rhio, the author of *Hooked on Raw,* explains why that occurs:

When you eat processed, enzyme-less foods, you put a heavy burden on your body, which then has to produce the enzymes missing in the food. One of the reasons you feel lethargic or sleepy after a cooked meal is because the body is diverting its energy to replacing the enzymes that were not supplied. By comparison, a raw food meal leaves you feeling light and full of energy. Uncooked foods are digested in one-third to one-half the time of cooked foods. The stress of creating and replacing enzymes meal after meal, day after day, year after year, greatly contributes to accelerated aging. Ingesting cooked food also causes the body to produce a surge of white blood cells (called leukocytosis). These cells normally defend against disease, infection and injury to the body, but their production is a routine effect of ingesting cooked foods as if the body considers such food a threat or danger. Leukocytosis does not occur when raw, unheated foods are eaten. Leukocytosis also occurs when additives, pesticides, and chemically based supplements are ingested.

On this healing diet, I strongly recommend that you find the freshest organic produce available to you. We frequently sprout alfalfa or other seeds to eat, recognizing that the freshest nutrients with the most enzyme potential are present in what is just in the process of sprouting in fresh water. I even start my sprouts in a strained seaweed sluice to provide higher iodine content. If you have a farmers' market close to your home, that produce would contain a higher quality of nutrients and enzymes than produce that has been shipped a greater distance. In fact, some would call food that has been shipped in from afar bathed or slathered in black oil, indicating the environmental costs—the so-called "carbon footprint"—incurred in transit. In his book *The Omnivore's Dilemma*, Michael Pollan states: "Today it takes seven to ten calories of fossil fuel energy to deliver one calorie of food energy to the American plate. The average distance that a food item travels is 1,500 miles [2413.5 km] to get to us." Enzyme depletion occurs in such lengthy transit time. Find garden-fresh organic produce options or a CSA if you can, to ensure that you are eating the freshest food available. In *The Macrobiotic Path to Total Health*, by Michio Kushi and Alex Jack, there is an interesting explanation for the creation of tumors in the body:

When the body loses the ability to create normal cells, tumors may arise, spread, and create a life-threatening condition. When the villi of the small intestine become coated with fat and mucus, they lose the ability to assist in the creation of healthy blood. Overworked lungs, kidneys, liver, and spleen will also weaken the blood and lead to the development of tumors. To protect the rest of the body from collapse, excess is localized in an isolated area that can be likened to a storage or toxic waste depot. When a particular storage site is full, another is created. In this way, tumors arise and metastasize throughout the body. Cancer is actually a wonderful self-defense mechanism by which the body protects itself from the effects of longtime dietary imbalance. If the excess were not isolated and contained, it would flood the bloodstream and cause death by blood poisoning (toxemia). Thus cancer is a healthy response to an unhealthy diet and lifestyle.

It postpones total collapse by several months or years. Cancer allows the person time to awaken to the underlying cause of his or her disease and, in most cases, to relieve it with proper diet and other natural means.

Our daily way of eating must be modified if illness is present so that what Kushi and Jack call "excess" is not allowed to be driven deeper into the body, where it can manifest in a more serious and life-threatening form. These deep diseases take longer to heal than do skin or blood disorders.

The Macrobiotic Path to Total Health also contains wisdom concerning the "macro-bios," called the "infinite life," a method to restore a person to health and happiness. Poor diet leads us to a type of detachment from the natural world. "Instead of taking responsibility and changing ourselves, we blame other people, society, nature, the universe, or God. Arrogance is both the last stage of sickness and the origin of all previous stages. It is the underlying cause of all sickness and unhappiness on our planet," the authors point out.

CHAPTER 6

Protein Facts and Fallacies

The truth is, Americans consume six to ten times as much protein as they need. That excess protein overworks the liver and kidneys, causing both these organs to become enlarged and injured. Excess protein consumption causes the kidneys to pull large quantities of calcium from the body, causing bones to weaken and kidney stones to form. Scientists have found that animal proteins are particularly damaging to the body, because so many of their amino acids contain sulfa, which is far more toxic to the liver and kidneys than vegetable proteins. One of the most time-honored approaches to healing the kidneys and liver, in fact, is to eat a low-protein diet, especially a diet low in animal proteins. When the protein content of the diet drops, kidneys are strengthened and very often healed. Americans have always had a love affair with animal protein— an affair that, unfortunately, is making us sick.

—JOHN A. MCDOUGALL, M.D., *THE MCDOUGALL DIET*

D r. McDougall further explains that "Protein is one of the most misunderstood and, consequently, most abused substances in the food supply. First, you should know that all plant foods contain protein. All of the protein you need and more can be easily derived from plant foods alone." Americans are consuming excessive animal protein. Not only do these proteins have little nutritional value, but excessive animal protein in the diet can cause serious health challenges due to the amount of sulfa that it contains. I have noted that only plants contain phytochemicals, which protect us from serious diseases. They also contain vitamins, minerals, fiber, protein, and antioxidants. It is protein that allows the plant to stand upright and gives it its structure. The only reason that animal foods contain minerals is that the animal eats mineral-rich plants.

Plant proteins are superior to animal protein because they are easier to digest and assimilate. Plants contain those eight essential amino acids in abundance, and by eating a variety of plants in your diet, you are assured that you will get 100 percent complete protein. The plant-based proteins are found inside fiber-dense plant cells. This fiber passes through our digestive system, providing us with healthy and regular bowel movements. Animal protein is inside of animal cells, the walls of which are constructed from cholesterol. Our digestive system is not well equipped to break down cholesterol. Meat constipates us, coats our stomach and intestines with grease and fats and cholesterol that is absorbed into our system makes our blood thick, clogs our arteries, and may eventually kill us, as it does many Americans. Just as enzymes and vitamins are destroyed by heat, amino acids are completely destroyed by heat above 160 degrees Fahrenheit (71°C). Cooking meats damages the meat proteins, causing the amino acid chains to congeal; these damaged proteins may be harmful to your body, causing inflammation in joints and tissue.

Another issue to consider is that excessive animal protein can harm your kidneys by making your system too acidic. The American Cancer Society conducted a ten-year study of 80,000 people trying to lose weight. The subjects who ate meat three times a week or more gained substantially more weight than those who avoided meat and consumed more vegetables. Further studies, published in the *Journal of Clinical Nutrition* and the *New England Journal of Medicine,* revealed that meat eaters are more likely to be less healthy and more likely to be overweight when compared to vegetarians.

The World Health Organization suggests that people should get only 5 percent of their calories from protein. Studies show that most vegan diets provide the ideal amounts of protein recommended by the WHO, while omnivores eat much more protein than the guidelines suggest. This may cause health risks, including a calcium imbalance that contributes to osteoporosis as well as compromised kidney function. This research indicates that too much protein can be dangerous to your health. The disease called gout is actually considered protein poisoning. The liver tries to break down excessive protein and makes uric acid and urea; since the kidneys cannot remove all that uric acid from the blood, it settles as crystals in areas where the blood flow is naturally slower, such as the toes. Bacteria enter these deposits and try to break them down. Unfortunately, these bacteria may then cause inflammation of cells and swelling.

If too much uric acid is generated, it may get deposited in the feet and hands, which would eventually cause gout. The least uric acid–forming foods are fresh produce, fruits, and vegetables. Another unfortunate side effect of excessive animal protein in the diet is related to the ingestion by the animal of toxic pesticides, herbicides, and added antibiotics (especially in cattle). I have had cases of women with bleeding nipples, hot flashes, and hormone imbalances due to excessive hormone-laden meat in their diet.

The world's longest research project concerning diet and heart disease, the Framington Heart Study, was launched in 1949. Dr. William Castelli, M.D., stated: "Vegetarians have the best diet. They have the lowest rates of coronary disease of any group in the country. Some people scoff at vegetarians, but they have a fraction of our heart attack rate and they have only 40 percent of our cancer rate. They outlive us."

John Robbins, author of *May All Be Fed,* goes further than specifying the advantages of vegetarianism in terms of longevity: "The real issue is quality of life. For a person who is not burdened by clogged and hardened arteries, whose kidneys and skeleton are not under siege from excess protein, and whose cells are not driven to cancerous multiplication by too much fat, the experience of life is thoroughly different from the experience of someone whose diet is based on animal products. The real advantage is not merely a matter of life extension numbers, but can be found in a body that remains strong and supple and a mind that remains clear and flexible as the years go by. A valid test to a good eating plan is the one that not only lengthens our lives, but allows us the great blessing of good health throughout the years."

So how do we measure appropriate amounts of protein in the diet? One way to consider protein consumption is by grams. On the average, a woman requires 46–50 grams of protein daily. Recent studies concerning nitrogen balance provide a more accurate way to determine the body's protein requirements. In his book *Eat to Live,* Joel Fuhrman, M.D., states that an easy way to calculate your own daily protein requirements is to multiply 0.36 grams by your body weight in pounds. For a 120-pound (55-kg) woman, that would translate into forty-three grams, and for a 150-pound (68-kg) male, that would be fifty-four grams. During pregnancy and breast-feeding, more protein is required. Athletes need to consume more calories, according to Ironman vegan athlete Dr. Ruth Heidrich. She discourages the use of protein supplements and stresses that if you want to build more muscle, "You have to overload it by putting more stress on it than it can handle. This is the ONLY way a muscle will get bigger and stronger." A diet that contains 12–15 percent protein is considered ideal for both strength and endurance athletes who consume a vegan diet. To athletes who want to keep their weight low, about 10–12 percent of calories as protein may be adequate. I suggest avocado and hemp protein shakes for athletes, as well as the addition of young coconut milk and the coconut pudding on the inside.

A vegan raw, plant-based diet includes plant sources such as sprouted seeds, grains, legumes, nuts, vegetables, and fruit. Plant protein is in no way inferior to animal protein, since it contains the same twenty-two amino acids as animal protein. Since complete protein building blocks contain twenty-two amino acids, the body has the ability to manufacture most of the amino acids it requires. Nine of the twenty-two—tryptophan, methionine, histidine, valine, phenyalanine, isoleucine, leucine, lysine, and threonine—are amino acids that must be obtained directly from the foods we eat. Quinoa is a grain that contains all these proteins, so it is called a complete protein food. Miso does as well. The other plant-based foods, like most whole grains, legumes, nuts, seeds, vegetables, and fruit, do not contain complete proteins by themselves. The body forms an amino acid pool throughout the day from the foods that we consume. The body can use gathered amino acids to make up complete protein. Nutritionists agree that if a person is eating adequate calories of plant-based foods, it is highly unlikely that he will be protein-deficient.

The average person in America consumes foods containing 120 grams of protein daily, mostly from animal sources. This puts a great stress on the kidneys and, as the nephrons in the filtering system deteriorate, it causes catastrophic premature aging of this important organ system. Excessive protein also causes bad breath, kidney stones, gout, osteoporosis, acid reflux, obesity, plaque retention in the arteries, elevated blood pressure, arthritis pain, and increased risk of cancer, especially colon cancer. Many people are addicted to the acids in meat and claim that they do not feel full after eating a plant-based diet. Given the risks involved in a high-protein diet, it is best to look at the research statistics before deciding that animal tissue protein is better than plant-based protein.

As reported in the May 2010 issue of the *American Journal of Clinical*

Nutrition, the participants in a seventy-four-week clinical trial who were on a low-fat vegan diet showed dramatic improvement when it came to four disease markers: kidney function, blood sugar control, cholesterol reduction, and weight control. This research is considered extremely important for diabetes research because previous studies collected data for six months or less. Also, as noted in the May 2010 edition of *Nutrition Reviews,* vegan and vegetarian diets were consistently associated with reduced rates of heart disease, diabetes, and obesity. Both of these studies were authored by Neal Barnard, M.D., David Jenkins, M.D., Ph.D., and other doctors and dietitians with the Washington Center for Clinical Research at George Washington University and the University of Toronto. Dr. Barnard shares this interesting fact: "A low-fat vegan diet has proved its staying power as one of the most effective long-term treatments for type 2 diabetes." We have to wonder why people who have diabetes are rarely given that beneficial information. There seems to be an unfortunate disconnect between research findings related to food consumption and health or disease consequences. When a patient visits a doctor's office, diet is rarely discussed. As I mentioned before, it is estimated that of the 125 medical schools in the United States, only 30 of them require their students to take a single course in nutrition. The average number of hours invested in nutrition education for the average American physician during four years of school is $2^1/_2$ hours. As a result, doctors are ill-equipped to give nutritional advice or implement educational programs for health, even though most modern illnesses are food- and lifestyle-related. The Himalayan Studies Research indicates that "Heart attacks are the most common cause of death in America, and it is the most preventable. A male meat eater has a 50 percent risk of a heart attack in his lifetime as opposed to 14 percent for the male vegetarian. Reducing intake of animal products reduces the risk by 90 percent." Whenever I suggest that a patient consider a plant-based diet, I often encounter resistance related to the overabundance of advertising misinformation.

As you check the protein content information below, you'll see that it is easy to consume more than enough protein from plant sources alone. Raw plant sources with bioavailable enzymes make the absorption of protein much easier. Some plant foods contain what are called *complete proteins.* This means they contain all of the essential amino acids that are considered to be the building blocks of all proteins. I always tell my patients who ask about getting enough protein in their raw diet to look at cows grazing in the field. They do not consume animal protein, yet they are much larger than we are. That cow is getting lots of energy and nutrients from the grass in the field. People who eat too much acidic meat find that they tend to become compulsive or addictive eaters who are never satisfied.

A medical research study, called the Oxford Vegetarian Study, has found that a properly balanced vegetarian diet is the healthiest diet of all. Over 11,000 volunteers participated in this study. For a period of fifteen years, researchers analyzed the effects that a vegetarian diet had on longevity, heart disease, cancer, and other diseases and disorders. The National Institutes of Health, in a study of 50,000 vegetarians, found that the vegetarians live longer and also have an impressively lower incidence of heart disease and a significantly lower rate of cancer than meat-eating Americans. And in 1961, the *Journal of the American Medical Association* reported that a vegetarian diet could prevent 90 to 97 percent of heart diseases.

The results of the consumption of meat studies from the Oxford Vegetarian Study stunned the researchers, but not as much as it did the meat industry: "Meat eaters are twice as likely to die from heart disease, have a 60 percent greater risk of dying from cancer and a 30 percent higher risk of death from other causes." The study also concluded that the incidence of obesity, a major risk factor for most diseases like type 2 (adult onset) diabetes, high blood pressure, and gallbladder disease, is much lower in people following a vegetarian diet. Americans of all age groups, races, and genders are getting fatter, according to a Johns Hopkins University research report. It is estimated that if the current trend continues, by 2014 one half of the American population will have diabetes.

A diet high in red meat seems to contribute to three forms of cancer: breast, prostate, and colon. In a study in Singapore, women were studied for breast cancer. It was determined that women who eat a Western diet with red meat increased their risk three times more than the women eating the typical regional vegan diet of northern China. Research has proven that diets high in red meat and low in green, leafy vegetables are associated with increased colon cancer risk. The body produces more acid when you eat meat because acid is used in the stomach to denature protein, and meat is a dense, protein-rich food. Proteins are long chains of amino acids that must be broken down into individual units of amino acids. Otherwise, they are too big to enter the bloodstream from the digestive system. *Denaturation* is the process of breaking down proteins into individual amino acids. When dense protein is denatured, the remaining long string of amino acids can be further broken down by enzymes in the small intestine. Eating meat increases the amount of hydrochloric acid your stomach must produce because hydrochloric acid is responsible for denaturing protein. Acidosis occurs when people eat a diet too high in acid-producing processed foods, like white flour, sugar, coffee, acid-forming drugs, chemical sweeteners, animal products including meat, and soft drinks. In addition, these same individuals consume far too little alkaline-producing foods like fresh vegetables and fruit. An acidic pH balance in the body will decrease the body's ability to absorb vitamins and minerals, decrease its ability to heal damaged cells, decrease the ability to detoxify heavy metals, allow tumor cells to grow, and make a person vulnerable to disease and fatigue. Even a slightly acidic blood pH of 6.9 may induce coma and death. If you want to restore yourself to health, your diet should consist of 80 percent alkaline-forming foods and 20 percent acid-forming foods. If the body is too acidic, it uses alkaline minerals to try to restore balance. If there are not enough minerals present, acids will build up in the cells. When food oxidizes in the body, it leaves a residue, or ash. If the residue minerals sodium, potassium, calcium, and magnesium predominate, they are designated as alkaline foods. The opposite of this is true if sulfur, phosphorus, chlorine, and incombustible organic acid carbon compounds predominate; the food is then designated as acidic. Alkaline foods include most leafy green vegetables, lentils, peas, sea vegetables, chlorella, cucumbers, seeds, nuts, garlic, onions, apples, avocado, green tea, and, surprisingly, lemons. Acid-forming foods include meat, fish, poultry, eggs, grains, and legumes.

A focus on protein in America borders on an obsession. Since World War II, the meat and dairy industries have spent billions of dollars promoting this obsession. Their influence begins in schools at the very early grades. Americans are taught that a meal is not a meal without meat and milk. Portion sizes of meat, chicken, or fish—often smothered in sauces or melted cheese—grew over the years, and one meal alone now comes close to fulfilling a day's worth of protein requirements.

There are far too many myths related to protein, and solid facts will reassure friends and family alike that a vegan diet is beneficial. Myths abound about the early meat-based diet of humans on this planet. It is documented that early humanoids were actually fruitarians. In 1979, Professor Alan Walker, a Johns Hopkins University paleoanthropologist, reported that preliminary studies of unmarked tooth enamel in early hominoids suggested that [our] prehuman ancestors apparently had a diet of mostly fruit.

Timothy Johns, Ph.D., a professor of human nutrition at McGill University, writes in *The Origins of Human Diet and Medicine:*

> Within the discussion of the diet of early humanoids, the question of the importance of meat versus plant-derived foods has continued to generate a debate with considerable philosophical, economic, political, and moral overtones. Not only what our ancestors ate but how they obtained it has important implications. The idea of "man the hunter" sustains an image of man as the dominant force in the biological world that is difficult to relinquish. In actuality, an emphasis on the hunting model in investigations of human subsistence is perhaps an artifact of the role of males in hunting and the social status attached to this activity. Dietary procurement is a fundamental determinant of biology, behavior, and social structure, and indeed has relevance for helping us understand human social relations. However, the incompleteness of the data and strong biases of various sides in the discussion combine to give us a cloudy picture.

Another bit of interesting information regards parasites. Research has shown that all meat eaters have worms and generally a high incidence of parasites in their intestines. This is hardly surprising since dead flesh is a favorite home for microorganisms of all sorts. A 1996 study by the U.S. Department of Agriculture confirmed that over 80 percent of ground beef is contaminated with disease-causing microbes from feces. The germs and parasites found in meat products weaken the immune system and can cause disease. Most food poisonings today are related to meat-eating or fecal contamination of foods. More than half a million Americans—most of them children—have been sickened by mutant fecal bacteria, *E. coli,* in meat. These germs are the leading cause of kidney failure among children in the United States.

People who feel concerned about protein intake on a raw vegan diet can rest assured that if they follow my 4-3-2-1 regimen, which offers the proper pH formula (your own fist-sized servings of 4 greens, 3 cruciferous vegetables, 2 fruits, 1 serving of nuts, seeds, or grains each day), they will receive more than adequate, safe protein in their diet. It is easier to eat too much protein than too little. One of my patients in her first appointment informed me that she ate red meat seven days a week and loved it. She was concerned because her cholesterol was high and her heart health was a major concern. After three years, she has eliminated most of the red meat from her diet, but it has not been easy for her. She was very aware that she was addicted to it. Recently, she voiced a concern that I have heard from many individuals who have consumed red meat on a regular basis. She said that no matter what she eats in the vegetable and fruit kingdoms, she is hungry in $2^1/_2$ hours. Meat sustains her and keeps her hunger at bay, she complained. I told her that hunger after $2^1/_2$ hours is the natural and healthy way to feel. Food that takes longer to digest is actually putrefying in the colon, rather than being digested and moving on at a healthy rate.

Table 6-1 shows the protein content of various vegetables, nuts, seeds, and grains. If you eat according to my 4-3-2-1 Raw Healing Diet, it is difficult not to get adequate protein on a daily basis. An average cup (200 ml) of raw vegetables may contain two grams of protein. One to two ounces (28–57 g) of nuts may contain fourteen grams of protein, the same as lean meat, fish, or chicken. We use nutritious hemp seeds instead of rice to accompany our raw stir-fry.

TABLE 6-1   PROTEIN CONTENT PER 100 GRAMS, OR 3.5 OUNCES

SEVERAL VEGETABLE SOURCES

Broccoli: 3 grams	Cabbage: 1 gram	Carrot: 0.5 gram
Celery: 1 gram	Cucumber: 0.5 gram	Spinach: 2 grams
Lettuce: 0.7 gram	Tomato: 2 grams	

SEVERAL BEAN OR LEGUME SOURCES

Dried beans: 21.4 grams	Lentils: 22–35 grams	Mung: 23.5 grams

SEVERAL NUT SOURCES

Almonds: 21 grams	Cashews: 20 grams	Brazil nuts: 14 grams
Pecans: 9 grams	Pine nuts: 14 grams	Walnuts: 6 grams

SEVERAL SEED SOURCES

Sesame seeds: 71.2 grams	Hemp seeds: 60–80 grams	Flax seeds: 25–30 grams

SEVERAL FRUIT SOURCES

Banana: 1.22 grams	Apple: 0.26 gram	Blueberries: 0.82 gram

Seeds are often overlooked in the American diet. Hempseed contains the highest concentration of essential fatty acids of any plant, and it contains all the essential amino acids necessary for a healthy life. As an added bonus, this complete protein is easily digested. We also use hempseed oil for salad dressings and in our smoothies. Both hemp and flax oil contain high levels of linoleic acid LA, which promotes immunity by retaining oxygen in the cell membrane, where it acts as a barrier to invading viruses and bacteria. Nutritionist Udo Erasmus, Ph.D., states, "Hemp butter puts our peanut butter to shame for nutritional value." Because it is so easily digested and assimilated, hempseed was once used to treat nutritional deficiencies brought on by tuberculosis.

CHAPTER 7

Education

Many of the major chronic diseases of modern industrialized societies, such as heart disease, hypertension, obesity, adult-onset diabetes, dental caries, and some types of cancer have a dietary basis.
—TIMOTHY JOHNS, PH.D., THE ORIGINS OF HUMAN DIET AND MEDICINE

I believe that Hippocrates said it best: "Let food be your medicine and medicine be your food." Why aren't Americans better informed about nutrition? Very few medical doctors learn about nutrition as part of their medical education. Funding from the pharmaceutical industry ensures that doctors learn to dispense drugs, rather than share dietary guidelines for health with their patients. Imagine what a different world this would be if only a minor percentage of the wealth from that industry was used to teach people how to eat better foods. Unfortunately, most schools of nutrition are supported by the industries that have a vested interest in their products. Children are taught the information provided by the Food and Drug Administration (FDA). The FDA gets much of its information from the food lobbies—a significant conflict of interest. Diabetes patients are provided with dietary guidelines issued by the dairy industry. I want you to know that I receive absolutely no kickbacks and have no industry support behind my years of research. The kale and romaine council are not paying me to share with you the value of dark leafy greens. I am giving you this information for educational purposes in hopes that you will do further research and, above all, avoid processed, dead foods. That being said, I would like you to know that I am sharing with you my own way of life. I'm not just lecturing about something I haven't tried myself.

One of my favorite stories is about a time when Mahatma Gandhi was asked by a mother to tell her child to stop eating sugar. He advised her to come back in a month. When they returned a month later, Gandhi stooped down, looked the child in the eyes, and simply said, "Please do not eat sugar. It isn't good for you." The mother asked Gandhi why he made her make such a long journey back for a message that he could have delivered a month ago. Gandhi smiled at her and responded, "Because a month ago I still ate sugar. Now I don't." As a vegetarian for thirty years, and a vegan for ten of those years, I have enjoyed extraordinary health most of my life, and especially since I have eliminated unnatural, enzyme-deprived, processed foods from my diet. Mostly, I eat a raw plant-based diet. Most days I feel like I am twenty, and believe me, twenty was decades ago. Even when discussing dietary lifestyles, we have opportunities to make poor or uneducated food choices. While a vegetarian diet may be healthy, over my years in practice, I have encountered some very sick vegetarians who ate a lot of cheese, chips, and cookies but no vegetables. Just choosing not to eat meat or animal products does not necessarily imply that you will make better food choices. One very vocal patient asserted that she would never attempt a vegetarian diet again. She was a vegetarian for three months and was constipated the entire time. Further in the interview, I learned that her vegetarian diet contained no vegetables whatsoever, but a lot of pizza, macaroni and cheese, chips, pasta, and doughnuts. She was choosing very poor options to replace meat indeed.

In a similar case, I was asked to discover why a child named Julia, in a vegetarian family of four, was always sick and cranky and misbehaved constantly. When I looked at her little face, I could see her "dairy shiners." She had black puffy bags beneath her eyes, almost as if she had been hit and suffered two black eyes. I learned that Julia craved and ate lots of potato and corn chips; processed dairy products derived from cows, including cheese sticks and American cheese slices, in particular; and suffered severe constipation. She also hated all vegetables except small carrots and all fruit except oranges. "Potato chip" vegetarians are all too common, and I consider this addictive behavior—feverish dairy and carbohydrate consumption—to be very unhealthy. Julia's case was not easy to counsel, since her mother was not at all motivated to wash vegetables, salad greens, or fruit. Her family ate mostly prepackaged, canned, bagged, and processed vegetarian foods that were loaded with high-fructose corn syrup, dairy, preservatives, and wheat gluten. Five days a week, Julia ate pasta with cheese on it. Her abdomen was always distended and I could tell that an inflammatory process was well underway in her colon. I suspected that she also was gluten-intolerant. After fielding several irate calls from her angry mother, stating that Julia's dairy-free dietary restrictions were just too difficult to maintain, I suggested that she and the entire family try my 4-3-2-1 Raw Foods Diet for just one week to see how well Julia would respond to it. Unfortunately, she never attempted to make it through even one day. A relative suggested that little Julia take a product to trick her system into believing that lactose could be tolerated so she could continue to eat the mac and cheese she loved. Sad but true. The consequences of such a forced remediation are that the body is tricked into tolerating a food that it cannot tolerate or readily digest on its own. Her body will suffer the consequences, whether Julia feels them or not. Many of the immune-compromised children I see in my practice do not like to eat vegetables, and their parents do not encourage them to do so. Green vegetables are natural detoxifiers and binders for toxic elements, especially since we have polluted air, water, and food to contend with in the twenty-first century. Without these binders, toxic debris settles in the system where you least want it to be.

I also have encountered individuals who are already on a raw vegan diet who have had severe health challenges related to unbalanced or poor food choices. Ironically, just as with faux-vegetarians, some of these raw cuisine adherents never eat real vegetables. They create exotic nut-mushroom "meats" (nut-based meat substitutes) and patés, plus date, nut, and cacao desserts and snacks, but all these dietary combinations are void of greens. Also present and problematic for these people may be pre-existing health zappers, such as parasites, yeast, miasms, and toxic metal retention that add to the toxic load. These people refused to be motivated to leave the body without binders, and to add to their diet the dark green vegetables that encourage their migration. Again, my raw, balanced pH approach helped these individuals to focus on providing the elemental needs of the body to first gently detoxify and then rebuild consistently, so the body could tolerate deeper detoxification efforts.

Even when we discuss food itself, we must recognize that it has changed over the past century. It is hard to believe that the pure food that sustained our hardy ancestors has been altered and is now virtually extinct. I shudder when I read the expression *conventional produce*. This is a label for nonorganic, pesticide–sprayed fruits and vegetables, or even genetically modified foods. It is scary to me that genetically modified foods have entered the market without labeling. People have no idea that what they are eating may be cloned or lacking the DNA of simple foods that they used to buy. It is just not the same type of food as it was ten years ago. There is nothing "conventional" about nonorganic food, and the label "conventional produce" misleads us to accept it as the norm. By the same token, after World War II, processed, prepackaged, and enriched food was considered to be far superior to whole foods. My grandmother told me that when she was a young woman it was frowned upon to feed your family whole foods. Fortunately, she did not embrace this philosophy. Processed foods and fast food are not good sources of sustenance for a healthy body.

When we wonder where nutrition education begins, often schools assume responsibility by providing age-appropriate materials for nutrition education. Unfortunately, they relinquish responsibility for this important educational experience to commercial interests. The dairy industry knows how to make money by spending money. It is one of the major contributors to school education programs. This seems like a conflict of interest to me. According to the Center for National Education Statistics, "Ninety-seven percent of schools report receiving nutrition lesson materials from at least one source outside the school, most often from professional or trade associations (87 percent) and the food industry (86 percent). However, for any given outside source, only 37 percent or less of schools used all or most of the materials received. Of the materials from sources outside the school, schools reported the highest classroom usage for those received from the food industry or commodities groups, professional or trade associations, the U.S. Department of Agriculture (USDA) Food and Nutrition Information Center, and state education agencies." While there has been concern about how dairy foods fuel childhood obesity, the dairy associations are leading the charge to ensure that milk consumption by students in schools increases rather than decreases. They are a large presence in most conferences concerning childhood obesity, including one recently hosted in New Jersey. Althea Zanecosky, M.S., R.D., representing the Mid-Atlantic Dairy Association and the American Dairy Association, said, "We work with schools throughout the state to provide nutrition education through a broad range of programs, ranging from classroom lessons to revamping cafeteria menus. Two years ago, we introduced a 'New Look of School Milk' in New Jersey cafeterias—a simple change in packaging from cardboard carton to a plastic jug—which resulted in an 18 percent average increase in milk consumption—and today over 414 schools in New Jersey have the 'New Milk.'"

In his book *May All Be Fed,* John Robbins relates the brainwashing process in the dairy industry's attempts to control the contemporary education of school-aged children:

In front of me is a coloring book found today in public schools. Purporting to teach children how to eat well, it has been supplied to school systems by the dairy industry. I know that it is representative of many of the 'nutritional education' materials used throughout the United States . . . Color Dad, it says. There are rules to follow:

1. If Dad drank milk today, we are to draw a "happy face." If he did not, then we are to draw a "sad face."

2. If he had ice cream today, we are to color his hair brown; if he did not, we are to color his hair blue.

3. If he had butter, we are to color his eyes blue. If he didn't have any butter, we are to color his eyes red.

4. If he had cheese, we are to color his face pink. If he didn't have any cheese, we are to color his face green.

You didn't (or don't as a child just learning) raise your hand and say, "Excuse me teacher, but I have some questions. What are the health consequences of eating a lot of milk, butter, ice cream, and cheese? Aren't these high in butterfat? And isn't butterfat a saturated fat? And don't dairy fats carry pesticide residues at very high levels of concentration? Who is it that profits from our believing that if we don't eat ice cream, butter, milk, and cheese, we end up looking terrible, with red eyes, a green face, and blue hair?"

I have had firsthand encounters with dairy industry–inspired "educational information." One of my first-grade patients' moms related how her daughter was in tears because she failed her nutrition test. Mom and her dairy-intolerant daughter had to visit the teacher that next day to discuss the information that was being tested. The teacher was understanding but inflexible. The children had to take the test at the end of the booklet and were graded on their correct regurgitation of the "facts." It seems that the child missed every one of them, and the teacher insisted that she correct her "errors." Mom maintained that her daughter's responses were absolutely correct and encouraged the teacher to look further for better educational materials. It seems that the school system insists that the school use materials supplied by the Dairy Council. Until our schools present nutritional information that is free of prejudice, our children will not learn the truth about good food.

My cancer patient agonized over the question of why she had not learned about good nutrition. When or where are we taught as parents or consumers to eat healthy foods? That question really deserves deeper reflection. The truth is we are primarily educated by the industries that promote polluted, altered, and processed foods. This industry and their research are not without bias. The next time that you see a milk mustache in a magazine advertisement, read the words that accompany the ad. It is not about all that superior calcium, as we were misled to believe. The ads now read that milk is a vital source of protein. No mention of calcium. Why? Because the calcium ads just weren't true. There is more bioavailable calcium in a spoonful of tiny sesame seeds than in a large glass of milk.

White bread is a denatured food from which over twenty vital nutrients have been removed. Only four chemical nutrients have been returned in a process called "enrichment." Organically grown fruits and vegetables contain more vitamins, minerals, and enzymes than "conventional" produce that is grown on depleted, chemically treated soils. Oftentimes, the growing time of vegetables for organic foods takes longer so there is more absorption of those vital vitamins and minerals. Most of the residues of toxic insecticides are systemic in the vegetables and fruit to which they are applied. When the American Cancer Society suggests that pesticides are acceptable as applied to our produce, they are creating the illusion that pesticides are not systemic or taken into the plant itself. They are absorbed by the produce. These toxins cannot be rinsed off. These toxic chemicals enter a fetus through the placenta. Recent research at Stanford Hospital found that the cord blood of newborns contained, on average, more than two hundred toxic chemicals. For future generations to be healthy, I feel that it is imperative for everyone, especially pregnant women and would-be mothers, to eat only organic, fresh, nutrient-rich foods.

In 1936, this expert testimony concerning soil mineral depletion was given to the Seventy-fourth Congress of the United States: "No man of today can eat enough fruits and vegetables to supply his system with the mineral salts he requires for perfect health." The use of commercial fertilizers, rather than traditional, natural methods of farming, was considered to blame for robbing the soil of nutrients and trace minerals needed to produce healthy plants for human consumption. To this day, industrial farming is perpetuating soil depletion. In his book *The Healing Power of Minerals,* Paul Bergner states that we cannot live healthy lives on the food of today. With that thought in mind, eating more raw fruits and vegetables optimizes assimilation of available nutrients, rather than further depleting our bodies of vitamins, minerals, and enzymes. It is the minerals in organic food that make it so tasty. If you are able to plant and grow your own organic vegetables and fruit, you are able to nurture and fertilize the plant yourself by providing natural sources of organic fertilizer to your soil. We use mineral-rich organic fertilizers, including mushroom base, to ensure there is adequate zinc, and we water our plants frequently with a sluice of seaweed water so iodine is available for them.

The industrialization of our society, with its subsequent pollution and enhanced food production, has allowed genetically modified (GMO), pesticide-infused, and cloned products to become a part of our own sensitive internal ecosystem. Xenotoxins and biohazards are known to cause disease and even death. Because moneyed food production and processing interests have been allowed to thrive, our own human bodies are paying an as-yet-undetermined high price. It is my belief that our health and even human DNA have been sacrificed to these polluting special industries. You do not have to research very far to find evidence that this is the case. As unfortunate as it is that Frankenfoods are legal in this country, it seems outrageous to me that advertisers of such nutrient-depleted foods target the young at a very early age, and parents are pressured to buy sugar- and sodium-laced dead GMO biohazards so their children will not feel left out. No wonder it is such a challenge to change bad food habits: there are so many addictions and emotions related to childhood consumption of processed foods. But this can be reversed through a process of alkalizing the body. Sugar, soda pop, and denatured grains are very acidic. Acids upset the pH and chemical balance of the body. As natural detoxifiers, greens are very alkaline and enzyme-rich.

ORAC UNITS

Your daily Oxygen Radical Absorbance Capacity (ORAC) score should be well over 5,000. In addition to understanding the recommended daily allowance of food and the pH of foods, potency tests for antioxidants in our foods have recently been developed. The scale of ORAC units, a measure of oxygen absorption, was developed by Dr. Guohua Cao, a chemist and physician at the National Institute on Aging in Baltimore. Dr. Cao, along with Dr. Ronald Prior of the Human Nutrition Research Center on Aging at Tufts University, established an ORAC score of 5,000 units daily to help prevent age-related diseases. The researchers were able to test the antioxidants in particular foods by placing them in a test tube to observe how long it took to destroy or neutralize the free radicals in each of the foods. They then assigned an ORAC score that corresponded to the free radical–destroying or –neutralizing power of that food. The hope for this research is that people will eat more fruits and vegetables, or at least focus on and consume those that have a higher ORAC score to prevent oxidative damage caused by free radical activity. The damage from these free radicals has been linked to early aging, cancer, and heart disease.

The measure of antioxidation for different densities of foods is based on the intake of 100-gram (g) servings. A denser food will generally weigh more and have a lower score. Table 7-1 is a list of fruits and vegetables that have a high ORAC score, measured per 100 grams. The raw diet transcends even ORAC units as a measure of health. If you are consuming a variety of fruits and vegetables, you are benefiting from a comprehensive and balanced daily diet of enzymes, vitamins, minerals, and the cofactors necessary for health and well-being.

TABLE 7-1   PRODUCE WITH HIGH ORAC UNIT SCORES

HIGH ORAC UNIT FRUITS

Prunes: 5,770	Pomegranates: 3,307	Raisins: 2,830
Blueberries: 2,400	Strawberries: 1,540	Raspberries: 1,220
Plums: 949	Oranges: 750	Grapes and cherries: 670

HIGH ORAC UNIT VEGETABLES

Kale: 1,770	Garlic clove: 1,662	Spinach: 1,260
Yellow squash: 1,150	Brussels Sprouts: 980	Alfalfa Sprouts: 930
Beets: 840	Avocado: 782	Red pepper: 710
Onion: 450	Corn: 400	Cauliflower: 385

The best ORAC values are found in deep-colored fruits and vegetables as well as green tea and oil-rich herbs like rosemary. Extra-virgin olive oil has the highest ORAC rating. If you add your ORAC units daily on your raw diet, you discover that you are taking great steps in delaying the aging process and the diseases that accompany it. But even more important, after three months you will feel years younger. Educate yourself about what good nutrition and healthy eating are all about, and then practice alkalinizing your body to create a healthier terrain for biochemical processes that prevent disease, mental disharmony, and premature aging.

BASIC VITAMIN AND MINERAL CONTENT
OF FRUITS AND VEGETABLES

There are twenty-two essential minerals for human nutrition. These are important components of body enzymes and facilitate proper bone, blood, and cellular function. The most important minerals are calcium, phosphorus, potassium, sodium, chloride, magnesium, and sulfur. The trace minerals include iron, iodine, zinc, chromium, vanadium, silicon, selenium, copper, fluoride, cobalt, molybdenum, manganese, tine, boron, and nickel. Plants absorb the inorganic earth minerals during their growth and bind them with living, organic molecules. Leafy greens are the best form of many minerals, especially when juiced.

Minerals

The following list contains natural sources of thirteen minerals, including trace minerals, and their plant-based source(s), plus symptoms of each mineral's deficiency.

Calcium: Mineral. RDA 1,500 milligrams (mg) daily to be used with 3 mg of boron and K_1. It is best consumed with magnesium-based foods. Sesame seeds, kale, collards, mustard greens, watercress, dark leafy greens, soybeans, asparagus, broccoli, figs. *Symptoms of deficiency:* Muscle spasms, bone loss.

Chromium: Trace mineral. RDA 400–600 mg daily. Broccoli, whole grains, corn, potatoes, mushrooms. *Symptoms of deficiency:* Metabolic syndrome, especially insulin resistance and maldigestion of fats, carbohydrates, and proteins.

Copper: Trace mineral. RDA 2 mg daily. Lentils and beans, whole grains, nuts, seeds, beets, avocados, radishes, leafy greens. *Symptoms of deficiency:* Nervous system disorder, inability to manufacture collagen, fatigue, baldness.

Iodine: Trace mineral. Sea vegetables. *Symptoms of deficiency:* Thyroid and endocrine disorders, including goiter. Delayed sexual development in children.

Iron: Trace mineral. RDA 25–35 mg daily. Leafy green vegetables, pumpkin seeds, potatoes, organic soybeans, whole grains, nuts, dates, peaches, pears, raisings, lentils, prunes, raisins, and sesame seeds.

Symptoms of deficiency: Anemia and paleness, fatigue, hair loss, nervousness, cracked lips.

Magnesium: Mineral. RDA 500–800 mg daily. Leafy greens, avocado, brown rice, bananas, apples, apricots, soybeans, broccoli, sesame seeds, lemons, potatoes, grapefruit, and beans. The fourth most abundant mineral in the body, 50 percent of total body magnesium is found in bone. Only 1 percent is found in blood, but it is essential because it is needed for more than three hundred biochemical reactions in the body, including regulating blood sugar levels and blood pressure. Magnesium is absorbed in the small intestines and excreted through the kidneys. *Symptoms of deficiency:* Irritability, sleep disturbances, muscle spasms, intestinal disorders, heart palpations or rapid heartbeat.

Manganese: Trace mineral. RDA 30 mg daily. Leafy greens, seeds, nuts, grains, tea, apples, apricots, grapefruit, cantaloupe, peaches, and figs. *Symptoms of deficiency:* Atherosclerosis, mental confusion, impaired hearing and vision, grinding of teeth, pancreatic issues, high blood pressure.

Molybdenum: Trace mineral. RDA 80 micrograms (mcg) daily. Leafy dark greens, beans, legumes, peas. *Symptoms of deficiency:* Impaired night vision, impotence in older males, increased heart and respiration rate, gum and mouth disorders.

Phosphorus: Mineral. RDA 1,200 mg daily. Beans, broccoli, grains, asparagus, corn, dried fruits, legumes, sesame, pumpkin, and sunflower seeds, and nuts. *Symptoms of deficiency:* Skin sensitivity, bone pain, fatigue and irritability, weak constitution.

Potassium: Trace mineral. RDA 3,500 mg. Dried apricots, sea vegetables especially dulse and kelp, chard, parsley, sunflower seeds, nuts, cauliflower, yams and potatoes, and dates. *Symptoms of deficiency:* Dry skin and acne, diarrhea, impaired mental, muscle spasms, heart arrhythmia, edema, insomnia, low blood pressure. A diet high in sodium and low in potassium has been linked to cardiovascular disease and cancer. A diet high in potassium and low in sodium protects against these diseases. Most people consume twice as much sodium as potassium. The healthy ratio should be a potassium to sodium ratio of 5:1.

Selenium: Mineral. RDA 400 mcg daily. Whole grains, Brazil nuts, onions, and vegetables. *Symptoms of deficiency:* Elevated cholesterol, cancer and heart disease, infections, fatigue, muscle weakness, and sterility.

Sodium: Trace mineral. RDA 2,400 mg daily. Cabbage, celery, grains. *Symptoms of deficiency:* Nausea, dehydration, low blood pressure, cramps, depression and confusion, heart palpations, inability to taste foods.

Zinc: Mineral. RDA 50 mg daily. Nuts, whole grains, beans, pumpkin and sunflower seeds. *Symptoms of deficiency:* Taste and smell deficiency. Eating disorders, thin nails, acne, hair loss, elevated cholesterol, impaired night vision, infections.

Fat-Soluble Vitamins, Measured in International Units (IU)

Vitamin A: RDA 10,000–50,000 IU daily. Yams, carrots, spinach, turnips, beet tops, mangoes, pumpkins, and yellow squash. Beta-carotene is a vitamin A precursor, converting to A in the liver as it is needed. Helps with anti-tumor immunity. *Symptoms of deficiency:* Constipation, nerve damage, five senses impairment, cancer, respiratory infection, and dry skin.

Vitamin D: RDA 1,000–2,000 IU daily. Mushrooms and sun exposure. I suggest supplementing. *Symptoms of deficiency:* Linked to cancer, psoriasis, weak muscles, tics, hypocalcemia, osteoporosis.

Vitamin E: 800–1,200 IU daily. Vegetable and nut oils, grains, and sunflower seeds. *Symptoms of deficiency:* Free radical damage, fibrocystic breasts, anemia, and some cancers.

Vitamin K: 150–200 mcg daily. Leafy dark greens, cauliflower, and broccoli. *Symptoms of deficiency:* Osteoporosis; bleeding issues, as it aids blood clotting. Vitamin K allows the osteocalcin molecule to bind with calcium to remain in the bone.

Water-Soluble Vitamins: B Vitamins and C in Mgs

B Vitamins

B_1 (thiamine): RDA 300 mg; B_2 (riboflavin): RDA 300 mg; B_3 (niacin): RDA 300 mg; B_5 (pantothenic acid): RDA 300 mg; B_6 (pyroxidine): RDA 2 mg; B_{12} (cyanocobalamin): RDA 500 mcg. B_{12} must generally be supplemented as it is rarely found in simple, unfortified plant sources except for sea vegetables and Brewer's yeast. Neither plants nor animals make vitamin B_{12}, as bacteria are responsible for producing vitamin B_{12}. Animals get their vitamin B_{12} from eating foods contaminated with vitamin B_{12} and then the animal becomes a source to provide vitamin B_{12} in the diet. Plant foods do not contain vitamin B_{12} except when they are contaminated by certain microorganisms or are fortified with vitamin B_{12}. Vegans need to consider fortified foods or supplements to get vitamin B_{12}.

Folic acid (and PABA): RDA 800–1,200 mcg daily. Of extreme importance during pregnancy.

Choline: (not always considered a vitamin, but is a B vitamin family member); works with Inositol): RDA 400–550 mg daily.

Inositol: RDA 250 mg. Most B vitamins are found in peas, dark and leafy greens including dandelions, nuts, beans and legumes, asparagus, corn, mushrooms, dates, sunflower seeds, squash, and tomatoes. *Symptoms of deficiency:* Fatigue, depression, sleep and digestive issues, headaches, inflammation, nerve disorders, anemia, tinnitus, pain and cramping, canker sores, edema, diarrhea, dizziness, poor digestion, and dermatitis. It can take up to five years for a deficiency to appear after the body is depleted of its stores.

Vitamin C

RDA 500–5,000 mg daily. (Sometimes taken to the level of bowel tolerance.) Red peppers, chilies, potatoes, dark leafy greens like kale and collards, oranges, broccoli, Brussels sprouts, avocados, asparagus, lemons, onions, radishes, strawberries, pink grapefruit, pineapple. *Symptoms of deficiency:* Infections, free radical damage and cancer, joint pain, bruising, fatigue, bleeding gums, scurvy. Excessive amounts at once can cause diarrhea.

ARE YOUR DAILY VITAMIN REQUIREMENTS BEING MET?

In 1981, 21,500 people were studied over a three-day period by the USDA. Not a single person consumed 100 percent of the RDA of all ten essential nutrients studied. Large numbers failed to consume 70 percent. Americans are literally starving from improper nutrition. It is estimated that, on a regular basis, 50 percent of Americans eat no fruit, and 25 percent eat no vegetables at all. Approximately 20 percent of their caloric intake is from refined sugars and sweeteners, 30 percent from refined grains, and 40 percent from fat. Many consume 10 percent from alcohol.

CHAPTER 8

What Are Good Foods?

*If your wealth is a number, your health would be the leading "1"
on a $1,000,000,000 ($1 trillion) jackpot. All the other zeroes
represent your material wealth—a house, a car, your investments,
family, friends, etc. As you can see, without the "1" in front, it will
just be $0,000,000,000 which is basically NOTHING. This is the
same as your health. If you're NOT healthy, if you're getting sick
all the time, all your riches do NOT matter.*

—ALLAN INOCENTE, *RICH MONEY HABITS*

I want to share with you my ultimate raw healing diet. This is a basic alkaline-pH diet that provides all the essentials for health and longevity, including the most important ingredient of all—enzymes. Most people who have followed this diet or, put better, established a new relationship with food claim that they have never felt better. The daily program is easy to follow. It is a ratio called 4-3-2-1, my raw foods diet for healthy eating. According to Dr. Bernard Jensen, in order to maintain a healthy pH, a person eating a healthy cooked diet should daily focus on eating six servings of vegetables, two servings of fruit, one serving of starch, and one serving of protein. For years, I educated students and patients about Jensen's theory of proper eating. While this method is acceptable if a person is relatively healthy, I find that we must be persistent and more assertive in our nutritional tactics if we are challenged by a health concern. My raw healing diet floods the body with enzymes to help the body heal diseased tissue and worn-out organs and organ systems. What is the 4-3-2-1 healing diet? This is a food formula that includes a base of 4 daily organic, raw servings of greens; 3 or more starchy, cruciferous vegetables that are not in the leafy first category of greens; 2 fruits; and 1 serving of high-protein whole grains, seeds, or nuts. A serving size is determined by the size of your own fist. I will give you further suggestions about this ratio of foods later on. Just remember that you are what you eat. So it is important to try to eat vegetables and fruits that are as fresh as possible. If you eat denatured processed, cooked, dead foods, you will feel dead. If you eat a lot of corn-fed animal protein and high-fructose corn syrup–laced soda pop, you may find your human tissue morphing into a corn chip. We Americans are, according to carbon-13 analysis, "corn chips walking." *The Omnivore's Dilemma* by Michael Pollan gives us a shocking analysis of the primary ingredient in most of our modern food. "There are some 45,000 items in the average American supermarket and more than a quarter of them now contain corn." If you eat living, enzyme-rich fruits and vegetables, you will feel alive and your body can heal more rapidly. Even if you are not on the ultimate healing diet, 75–80 percent of your diet should consist of vegetables and fruits in their natural, uncooked state. Remember the reaction in the body to cooked food is called leukocytosis. Food is viewed skeptically by the body as a foreign invader. The body wants to attack this invader, and over the years of only eating processed, cooked foods, the body may eventually attack the cells of the body itself, since it cannot isolate the true invader. This cellular affront marks the beginning of an autoimmune disorder.

It is useful to think in terms of good foods replacing dead foods in your daily diet. One of my favorite greens is alfalfa sprouts. We also add dry nutritional alfalfa powder to our daily smoothies. Alfalfa is one of the richest sources of protein, containing 18.9 percent. Wheat contains 13.8 percent, beef 16.5 percent, and milk only 3.3 percent. An acre of alfalfa can contain as much as 1,200 to 1,400 pounds (545–636 kg) of protein. Soybeans on the same land can yield 700 pounds (318 kg) of protein. We eat at least a cup (200 ml) of alfalfa sprouts daily. They are fresh and loaded with enzymes. Besides its protein-rich nature, alfalfa is also a great source of iron, plus vitamins A, K, C, and B, especially B_6. If you live in a city or a polluted area, alfalfa could help your body to cope with the daily assault of chemical or environmental toxins.

Cauliflower is one of those superfoods that is essential in a raw healing diet. It is a good source of protein, thiamine, riboflavin, niacin, magnesium, and phosphorus, and a very good source of dietary fiber, vitamin C, vitamin K, vitamin B_6, folate, and pantothenic acid, potassium, and manganese. Folate prevents anemia, cancer and heart disease. Just four little florets of cauliflower a day will provide most of our daily vitamin C requirements. Throw those into a raw stir-fry or top a salad with cauliflower.

FATS AND OILS

Oils are important to consider in a raw healing diet. There has been much misinformation considering various oils in the past. If you follow the misinformation, you will often find a conflict of interest in the research. In other words, researchers are often paid by producers to malign competing products. For example, coconut oil was misrepresented by the commercial American soybean and corn oil industry as being an artery clogger. What was not reported was that hydrogenated coconut oil was used in the studies instead of the virgin coconut oil used for centuries as a staple food. We now know that hydrogenation, which involves artificially adding a hydrogen molecule to oils in order to ensure that they have a longer shelf life, creates the problem, not coconut oil itself. In fact, in its virgin form, coconut oil is one of the most stable oils you can buy. Hydrogenated soy, corn, and canola oils are packed with dangerous transfats and processed with toxic hexane solvents. These dangerous oils are routinely added to packaged foods. Hydrogenation has added inches to waistlines and is now linked with numerous health-threatening diseases. This misinformation concerning coconut oil was adopted by many heart-smart cookbooks. The message, while unsubstantiated, was clear: Avoid coconut oil. The poor countries that produced coconut oil could not fight the entrenched American grain and food industry. For more information, refer to *The Healing Miracles of Coconut Oil* by Bruce Fife, N.D. In it, Fife explains some alarming facts: "In India, within a year of switching from coconut oil to partially hydrogenated soybean oil, the number of deaths due to heart disease tripled. Researchers estimate that over 30,000 premature deaths in this country are due to partially hydrogenated oils." He goes on to explain the benefits of coconut oil: "Fifty percent of coconut oil is laurel acid. The only other good source of lauric acid is mother's milk." Three to four tablespoons (45–60 ml) of coconut oil daily are useful.

Dr. Mary Enig, one of the leading authorities on fats, tells us more about lauric acid:

Approximately 50 percent of the fatty acids in coconut fat are lauric acid.

Lauric acid is a medium-chain fatty acid, which has the additional beneficial function of being formed into monolaurin in the human or animal body. Monolaurin is the antiviral, antibacterial, and antiprotozoal monoglyceride used by the human or animal to destroy lipid-coated viruses such as HIV, herpes, cytomegalovirus, influenza, various pathogenic bacteria, including listeria monocytogenes and heliobacter pylori, and protozoa, such as giardia lamblia. Some studies have also shown some antimicrobial effects of the free lauric acid.

Let's take a look at the healing properties of coconut oil: it is antiviral, antifungal, and antibacterial. It attacks and kills viruses that even have a lipid coating, such as herpes, HIV, hepatitis C, the flu, and mononucleosis. It kills bacteria that causes pneumonia, sore throats, cavities, urinary tract infections, meningitis, and food poisoning. As an antifungal, it kills yeast infections, including candida, ringworm, thrush, diaper rash, and athlete's foot. It helps the body heal faster and supports immune function, protecting us from a variety of cancers. It reduces the symptoms of types 1 and 2 diabetes by bolstering the body's use of blood glucose. It assists the heart by preventing blood platelets from sticking together and creating clots. As a medium-chain fatty acid, it is broken down quickly and provides quick energy. Applied to the skin, it forms a barrier against infections and protects us from damaging UV rays.

In his book *Healing with Whole Foods,* Paul Pitchford states: "Plants that grow in cold climates are relatively more concentrated in omega-3s. These include hard red winter wheat and cold-climate nuts, seeds, grains, and legumes. Omega-3s are sometimes compared with anti-freeze, since they keep the blood relatively thin in cold weather, yet a number of clinical trials indicate omega-3s never cause or provoke hemorrhage." Population studies indicate that people who consume a diet rich in omega-3 oils have a significantly reduced risk of developing heart disease. Omega-3 fatty acids lower levels of fibrinogen, which is a soluble plasma glycoprotein that is converted by thrombin into congestive fibrin during blood coagulation, LDL cholesterol, and triglycerides, and inhibits excessive platelet aggregation. Omega-3s also lower blood pressure when it is high.

Udo Erasmus, Ph.D., has written an informative book called *Fats that Heal, Fats That Kill.* He explains that omega-9 fats are found in large quantities in olive, almond, avocado, peanut, pecan, cashew, filbert, and macadamia oils. He states: "GLA is a special type of omega-6 that provides benefit for arthritis and premenstrual syndrome. As much as 10 to 25 percent of affluent societies could benefit from its use. Under certain circumstances of illness and dietary deficiency, our body may be unable to make GLA from omega-6 and Evening Primrose Oil can compensate for this inability." Borage and black current oils are two other GLA-containing oils. Eczema responds positively to GLA supplementation. Erasmus explains that omega-3s are useful in treating skin problems like hives and psoriasis, but also can heal a plethora of other diseases: osteoarthritis and rheumatoid arthritis, kidney disease, ulcerative colitis, depression, bronchial asthma, enlarged prostate, and migraine headaches.

Flax could be dubbed the "forgotten oil" because manufacturers have found nutritious oils to be less profitable. The vital nutrients and essential fatty acids that give flax its nutritional benefits also give it a short shelf life, making it expensive to produce, store, and transport. Yet those who are nutritionally aware continue to rank flax high on the list of important foods. Because of recent scientific studies validating the health benefits of omega-3 fatty acids, flax oil has graduated to a status of health and scientific respectability. You can enjoy a tablespoon (15 ml) of flax oil or its equivalent of two tablespoons (30 ml) of freshly ground flaxseed meal. It is the best source of omega-3s and a good source of omega-6, or linoleic acid (LA). Sunflower, safflower, and sesame oil are greater sources of omega-6 fatty acids, but they are void of any omega-3 fatty acids. Flax oil consists of approximately 45–60 percent of the omega-3 fatty acid alpha-linolenic acid (ALA). These two essential fatty acids cannot be created in the human body and must be obtained from the diet. These vital essential fatty acids provide energy. The highest-lignan flax oil is a source of lignans, which are phytochemicals that boost immunity. In addition to nutritious fats, flax seeds contain other nutrients and fiber that actually make eating the whole seed better than consuming just the extracted oil. The healing attributes of flax involve soothing the digestive tract and as a treatment for constipation. A decoction (created by mixing the seeds with hot water and let soak for about 10 minutes) can prove to be soothing to the digestive tract and can also be used to treat respiratory and urinary disorders. The traditional use of flax for constipation is to eat one to two tablespoons (15–30 ml) of soaked or ground whole seeds with plenty of water. The seeds swell up in the intestines and encourage bowel movements. DHA is a special type of brain-feeding oil that is an omega-3 fatty acid found in fish oil; most people are not aware that DHA and eicosapentaenoic acid (EPA) can also be found in certain brown and green algaes that are eaten by fish.

Olive oil is also a heart-healthy, 80 percent–monounsaturated oil. It has a high concentration of fatty acids: studies indicate fatty acids promote "good" cholesterol (HDL) while lowering "bad" cholesterol (LDL.) Polyunsaturated fatty acids lower both LDL and HDL levels in the blood, but they do not affect their ratio of one to the other. Monounsaturated fatty acids, like those in olive oil, are able to control LDL levels while raising HDL levels. No other naturally produced oil has as large a proportion of monounsaturated fatty acids as olive oil, which contains oleic acid. The modest amount of well-balanced polyunsaturated fatty acids that are found in olive oil are well-protected by antioxidant substances. Since only saturated, animal-derived foods contain cholesterol, olive oil is cholesterol-free. Cholesterol is not entirely harmful; it is an essential building block for cell membranes, nerve fiber coverings, vitamin D, and sex hormones. The liver manufactures all the cholesterol it needs, so any cholesterol in foods we eat adds to that amount and becomes an excess. Excess cholesterol causes an accumulation of fat deposits, known as plaque, along the walls of blood vessels. This plaque builds up over time, narrowing the arteries, and then reducing blood flow. Animal cholesterol increases the risk of heart attacks and strokes. Good-quality olive oil contains substantial vitamins and nutrients, like vitamins A, B_1, B_2, C, D, E, and K, plus iron. The powerful antioxidants like vitamins E and K, and the polyphenols found in olive oil, provide a defense mechanism to help protect the body from cancer, inflammation, and liver disorders. Olive oil is also known to be gentle on the digestive system and even may help to prevent constipation, gallstones, ulcers, and gastritis; treat urinary tract infections; and soothe ulcers. Olive oil accelerates brain development and also strengthens bones. Olive oil has a reputation for delaying the aging process.

Avocados have 3.5 grams (g) of unsaturated fat, which is important for normal growth and development of the central nervous system. This makes avocados one of the first fresh fruits a baby can enjoy. It is sodium- and cholesterol-free, and it contains nearly twenty vitamins, minerals, and phytonutrients (nutrients that prevent chronic diseases), including 8 percent of the recommended daily value of folate; 4 percent daily value for fiber and potassium; 4 percent daily value for vitamins C and E, fiber, and potassium; and 2 percent of the daily value for iron. A serving also contains eighty-one micrograms of the carotenoid lutein and nineteen micrograms of beta-carotene. The avocado is virtually the only fruit that has monounsaturated fat. Avocados have also received a bad rap as being a fatty food, but the opposite is actually true. Avocados are encouraged in a heart-healthy diet as well as for healthy weight loss.

GARLIC AND ONIONS

Onions and garlic are members of the lily family, as are leeks, chives, scallions, and shallots. They are characterized by their rich content of thiosulfinates, sulfides, sulfoxides, and other somewhat strong-smelling sulfur compounds. In onions, the cysteine sulfoxides are primarily responsible for the distinctive flavor, and the thiosulfinates have antimicrobial properties. Onion works effectively against many bacteria, including *Bacillus subtilis, Salmonella,* and *E. coli.* Onion is not as powerful as garlic, since garlic has about four times the sulfur compounds found in onion. Onions have a variety of medicinal effects. In traditional Chinese medicine, onions are used to treat such diseases as angina, coughs, bacterial infections, and breathing problems. The World Health Organization suggests using onions for the treatment of poor appetite and also to prevent atherosclerosis, as well as using onion extracts to treat asthma, coughs and colds, and bronchitis. Onions alleviate bronchial spasms. An onion extract was found to decrease allergy-induced bronchial constriction in asthma patients as well as increase growth of friendly flora in the gut. In addition, onions can reduce the risk of tumors developing in the colon. The sulfides in onions are similar to those found in garlic, which may lower blood lipids and blood pressure. Onions also have substances that promote fibrinolytic activity, that is, suppressing platelet clumping, and they are natural anticlotting agents. Rich in a variety of sulfides, onions provide some protection against tumor growth. In central Georgia, where Vidalia onions are grown, mortality rates from stomach cancer are about one-half the average level for the entire United States. Chinese people tend to have a 40 percent lower risk of stomach cancer because they have the highest intake of onions, garlic, and other lily-family vegetables.

Garlic's benefits include lowering bad cholesterol and blood pressure, aiding circulation, and preventing stroke. It contains vitamins C and B_6, selenium, magnesium, potassium, calcium, manganese, and flavonoids. Garlic has been used as a natural cure for common ailments, such as acne, colds and flu, herpes, and wrinkles because of its natural antioxidant and antibacterial, antiviral, and antifungal properties. If you wish to further detoxify, you might consider crushing a clove or two of garlic into lukewarm water, straining, and drinking the liquid twice a day. Be careful not to do this on an empty stomach if you are sensitive to garlic. This detox is also good for the pain associated with arthritis and asthma attacks, because the sulfur compounds in garlic have been found to have anti-inflammatory effects by inhibiting the activity of inflammatory enzymes. Cut garlic can be applied directly to the skin as a remedy for acne or herpes. Vitamin C also increases body oxygen levels and interferon production, which are both good for treating herpes.

Population studies have demonstrated that eating garlic on a regular basis—along with onions, chives, and scallions—can reduce the risk of esophageal, colon, and stomach cancer because it reduces the formation of carcinogenic compounds. In animal laboratory studies, garlic's sulfur compounds have been found to stop the growth of various cancers, including skin, stomach, colon, breast, and oral cancer. Garlic also contains the antioxidant selenium, which is well-known for its anticancer properties. Selenium is used by our bodies to produce glutathione peroxidase. Glutathione is a powerful antioxidant that may be useful in the management of some cancers, atherosclerosis, diabetes, lung disorders, problems associated with noise-induced hearing loss, male infertility, and to prevent toxic fluid buildup in the body. It may also have some antiviral activity and has been used to treat AIDS. Selenium supplements are often recommended for the treatment and prevention of herpes. Selenium is also found in Brazil nuts. Some of the degenerative effects of diabetes, such as diseases of the kidney, retina, and nervous system, may be prevented by garlic.

Raw Onion Remedies

One of the remedies that I suggest for patients over two years old who have cough, colds, or upper-respiratory infections is to add a minced clove of garlic to a tablespoon (15 ml) of raw or regular honey twice a day. They should take this between meals in amounts appropriate to their age. An adult would take the entire tablespoon, but children would take perhaps half or less, according to their age.

Onion has been used externally as a salve for the treatment of burns, abrasions, skin inflammations, wounds, ulcers, and eczema. Internally (one to two grams of dried herb daily), it has been used for colitis, gastritis, and bleeding duodenal ulcers. Recent research proves its efficacy in the prevention and treatment of radiation burns.

Onion has also been employed by moms and dads as a home remedy for ear pain and healing. They might put half a small onion in the blender with a tablespoon (15 ml) of water and pulse it until it is like soup. Strain this in a coffee filter, and then add a couple of tablespoons (about 30 ml) of olive oil to the strained onion drippings. The onion acts as a pain reliever and has qualities like an antibiotic. Put this in a bottle with a dropper and put a few warmed drops in the ear. It is best to turn the dropper vial upside down in hot water to warm the oil; never put herbs, teas, or oils in the microwave to heat. Test for warmth on your wrist first.

HELPFUL VITAMIN SUPPLEMENTS
TO HELP YOUR TRANSITION TO RAW

Many people may need to supplement their diet according to their lifestyle or health concerns. If you suffer from a stressful lifestyle, you may wish to consider the addition of B vitamins with food (especially B_6 and B_{12}, or biotin, if you have blood sugar issues) and an adrenal support tea like licorice (if your blood pressure is not elevated) or panax ginseng. A calming tea, like chamomile or valerian, could replace a cup of coffee to soothe anxiety. Dandelion leaf tea is high in potassium and is one of my favorites. It acts as a bitter in the body that thins the bile in the gallbladder and liver. If taken before meals, it also functions as a natural diuretic. If you have osteoporosis, I never suggest supplementing with calcium, since that stresses the kidneys and the unabsorbed extra calcium may adhere to the joints or combine with lactic acid to cause crunchy calcium deposits in the muscles. I am shocked that doctors are still recommending a calcium carbonate stomach anti-acid product containing aluminum (yes, it is naturally occurring, but all aluminum has been implicated in Alzheimer's disease). Another common doctor-prescribed calcium product contains titanium dioxide, a known carcinogen. If you eat greens daily, as you should, a calcium deficiency is generally not an issue, unless you have high blood pressure, migraines, or muscle cramps. In such a case, supplementing with 750 milligrams (mg) of calcium glycinate might be helpful. A lack of bone-building walking or other forms of aerobic exercise, and/or a deficiency of vitamins K and D or boron, may be the root cause of osteoporosis or osteopenia. If you live in a place where you do not receive enough sunlight November through May, new research indicates that the addition of 3,000 IU of vitamin D daily may help to prevent cancer. Many people who do not eat magnesium-rich foods generally have a magnesium deficiency. I tell my patients that I am more concerned about a magnesium deficiency, which can cause heart palpitations, than I am calcium deficiency. Magnesium helps over three hundred enzymes to function in the body. These functions include muscle activity and metabolism. Fibromyalgia and chronic muscle pain are associated with magnesium deficiency. If you are trying to lose weight, magnesium is essential. Iodine is not present in a useful amount in most people's daily diets unless you eat sea vegetables. Since we have so many thyroid issues in America, I suggest the addition of one tablespoon (15 ml) of sea vegetables or a liquid iodine supplement.

Early on, I recommend to my patients a professional multivitamin (that is, a high-potency liquid multivitamin sold by health care professionals). The reason I do this is that many are not able to either digest or absorb the nutrients in a tablet or capsule. If you have a funny feeling in your chest near the sternum, you have an inflammation near the pyloric valve that could lead to a hiatal hernia. Pills actually can get stuck there. If that is the case, four ounces (113 g) of aloe vera juice prior to taking the pills may be useful. To the Aqueous Multi Plus vitamin, I add liquid vitamins B_{12}, D, A, and E, together with zinc, magnesium, iodine, and liquid amino acids. Research in the past into vitamins A and E has cast aspersions on these supplements, and as a result, many people avoid them, not sure what to take and when to take it. Vitamin E is important in the formation of red blood cells and it helps the body to use vitamin K to prevent osteoporosis. People who cannot absorb fat properly generally develop a vitamin E deficiency, which may lead to loss of muscle mass and muscle weakness, unsteady gait, impaired vision, and abnormal eye movements. Chronic deficiency of vitamin E may cause kidney and liver problems. Population studies show that the antioxidants in vitamin E may lower the risk of heart disease. The recommended dose of vitamin E is 400 IU of d-alpha tocopherol.

If you are able to digest and absorb nutrients, take a high-quality raw multivitamin that is available in most health foods stores. Make sure that you are receiving D, B_{12}, B_6, magnesium (400 mg daily if you are stressed), and iodine in the multivitamin. Most of the hard-shelled, drugstore variety vitamins are not broken down in the digestive system; they're propelled through the digestive system and preserved until eliminated in their original state. Avoid supplements with fillers like silica that stress the kidneys or that contain titanium dioxide, a known carcinogen.

Minerals in plants are much more bioavailable and, since they are mixed with organic molecules, are present in the living form rather than lifeless. Most mineral supplements are lifeless and may cause problems for the kidneys or in the body if they are overconsumed. If calcium is in the carbonate form, it is difficult for that larger molecule to pass through the permeable tissues, and its accumulation may cause kidney stones or lodge in the feet or joints. The big seven, or major, minerals include magnesium, potassium, calcium, sodium, phosphorus, chloride, and sulfur. The trace or minor minerals are iodine, iron, zinc, copper, selenium, molybdenum, boron, nickel, manganese, tin, chromium, vanadium, silicon, fluoride, and cobalt. In studying environmental allergies, I have found a missing link for patients who have a deficiency in molybdenum. Research indicates that high-sodium, low-potassium, junk-food diets are promoting cancer and cardiovascular diseases, including strokes, elevated blood pressure, and heart disease. Fresh fruits and vegetables are potassium-rich and low in sodium. Potassium is an important electrolyte that works with the kidneys to control fluid volume and distribution, as well as promoting stress reduction, adrenal, heart, and muscle health. Dulse, my favorite sea vegetable, is not only rich in iodine, it has over 8,000 milligrams of potassium per half cup. For that reason, I suggest that the salt shaker be replaced by the ground dulse shaker. Kelp is also rich in potassium, as are dark green leafy vegetables.

Please read Chapter 3 on foods and their vitamin content to clarify what to eat each day to promote the body's health. Remember that the state of the small intestine is vital to the absorption of vitamins and minerals. L-Glutamine and bromelain, taken between meals, are extremely important in healing inflammation in the small intestines.

RECOMMENDED DAILY ALLOWANCE OR UNITS FOR HEALTH

When I teach nutrition classes, I am always careful to note how research has proven that what was once considered to be the recommended daily allowance of vitamins daily was and is insufficient to support a healthy body. The FDA's Food Pyramid has been modified so much that it is confusing at best. Even Harvard Medical School points out that it fails miserably as a model for better nutritional understanding for Americans. They state: "We can't look at a pyramid these days without thinking of food and healthy eating. There was the U.S. government's Food Guide Pyramid, followed by its replacement, My Pyramid, which is basically the same thing only pitched on its side. The problem was that these efforts have been quite flawed at actually showing people what makes up a healthy diet. Why? Their recommendations have been based on out-of-date science and influenced by people with business interests in their messages." I feel that the vertical pyramid provides enough uncertainty to keep people from understanding what good nutrition is. I will share what Harvard researchers, who accept no subsidized funding, feel is important to understand about nutrition. They call this "Five Quick Tips for Following the Healthy Eating Pyramid":

1. Start with exercise. A healthy diet is built on a base of regular exercise, which keeps calories in balance and weight in check.

2. Focus on food, not grams. The Healthy Eating Pyramid doesn't worry about specific servings or grams of food, so neither should you. It's a simple, general guide to how you should eat when you eat.

3. Go with plants. Eating a plant-based diet is healthiest. Choose plenty of vegetables, fruits, whole grains, and healthy fats, like olive oil. (*Note:* I suggest that you avoid canola oil, due to its broad genetic modification.)

4. Cut way back on American staples. Red meat, refined grains, potatoes, sugary drinks, and salty snacks are all part of American culture, but they're also terribly unhealthy. Go for a plant-based diet rich in nonstarchy vegetables, fruits, and whole grains. And if you eat meat, fish and poultry are the best choices.

5. Take a multivitamin, and maybe have a drink. Taking a multivitamin can be a good nutrition insurance policy. Moderate drinking for many people can have real health benefits, but it's not for everyone. Those who don't drink shouldn't feel that they need to start.

For further information, please see The Nutrition Source, Department of Nutrition, Harvard School of Public Health, www.thenutritionsource.org, and *Eat, Drink, and Be Healthy,* by Walter C. Willett, M.D., and Patrick J. Skerrett.

CHAPTER 9

What Is Not Raw

> *Nothing will benefit human health and increase the*
> *chances for survival of life on Earth as much*
> *as the evolution to a vegetarian diet.*
>
> —ALBERT EINSTEIN ON DIETARY CHOICES

Here is an important list to help you know what is *not* raw. I feel that it might be useful for you.

Following are some interesting questions that I have been asked about the raw/not raw diet dilemma and my responses. Some seem like sensible questions; others contain a hint of self-sabotage or desire to defend the old pattern of destructive eating habits.

WHAT IS NOT RAW?	
QUESTION	ANSWER
Can I drink beer or wine while on a raw diet?	No. Drink tea, water, and organic coffee in moderation.
Can I eat chicken or fish?	No. You might try the recipe "Not the Chicken, or Not the Tuna" recipes. Tuna uses kelp; chicken, poultry seasoning.
Can I eat chocolate or candy?	No. Try raw cacao for chocolate and date cookies.
Can I eat sugar or artificial sweeteners?	No. Try raw agave nectar, raw honey, or stevia.

Can I drink milk on a raw diet?	No. Not unless it comes from a young coconut.
Can I eat cheese or eggs?	No. See recipes for raw cheese. It is yummy.
Can I eat cow dairy ice cream?	No. Try recipes for ice cream made from coconut, hemp, or fruit smoothies instead.
Can I eat oatmeal for breakfast?	No. Try raw granola.
Can I eat steak or hamburger?	No. Try marinated portabella mushroom or raw nut patés instead.
Can I eat potato chips?	No. These are fried or baked. Try nori or celery for the crunch.
Can I eat popcorn?	Not recommended. If you do, do so in moderation with sea salt or nutritional yeast only.
Can I eat pie?	Not unless it is raw. There are lots of recipes for raw pie, including creamy, pudding-like, or crunchy fruit varieties.
Can I eat bread, toast, or pancakes?	No. There are raw bread recipes, and many people enjoy raw crackers that you can buy or make. My favorite is a raw onion bread recipe. Also there are recipes for raw pancakes.
How can I eat at a restaurant?	Order a great salad or a side of raw veggies from the menu. Try for organic whenever possible.
Can I eat bottled salad dressing?	No. See any of the recipes in this book. If you are at a restaurant, ask for a vinaigrette or ask for olive oil and a slice of lemon.
Can I eat jams or jellies?	No. Make a raw version for your raw bread or crackers.
What can I eat for a snack?	Try apples or celery filled with almond butter and sprinkled with cinnamon or raisins. If you crave sweets, try a "Selenium Hot Dog" (see page 249) or a raw pear or raspberries.

AVOID THE FOLLOWING—IT IS NOT RAW VEGAN

The following list will help you better understand what is not raw vegan and should be avoided while on the 4-3-2-1 Raw Healing Diet. If in doubt, don't buy or eat it.

Food in a can: It has been cooked to a certain temperature to seal and preserve.

Food in a box: Read the ingredients. Most boxed foods are processed, denatured food.

Food in a jar: It has been cooked to seal and preserve. There are a few raw foods in a jar, like honey, miso, and agave, and raw nut butters, such as almond, sunflower, and cashew. These are the exceptions.

Food in a package: Check the label. Some raw food manufacturers are now sealing their raw foods in cellophane packages, but the label must indicate that it is raw.

Precooked foods: Those that have been cooked over 115 degrees Fahrenheit (46°C).

Dairy products: While there is some unpasteurized "raw" dairy, it is not vegan.

Cheese is also not raw. There are recipes for raw vegan cheese often made from pine nuts or cashews, so don't be confused if you see it in a recipe.

Baked goods: Most have been baked in an oven over 115 degrees (46°C) and contain denatured flours, eggs, and dairy.

Eggs: They are generally cooked and are not vegan.

Condiments: These are cooked over 115 degrees (46°C) to seal and preserve them. Ketchup is not raw.

Sauces: Soy sauce is not raw. Bragg Aminos or Nama Shoyu is okay, but use sparingly.

Table salt: Most is made from chemicals with iodine added. Sea salt is okay.

Flours or oatmeal: Only "groats" or the raw seed of either is acceptable.

Seasonings: Raw fresh is best. Some recipes call for simple dried herbs and you can use these to enhance recipes. Try to use only organic or fresh whenever possible.

Lemon or lime juice in a bottle: These are not raw. Try to use the real thing.

Meat: Fish, beef, pork, lamb, turkey, and chicken of any preparation is not part of this diet.

Soda pop or any canned or bottled beverages: None of these, including the fruit smoothie types, are on this diet.

WHAT IS RAW VEGAN AND CAN IT BE USED

The following list may be helpful for you to understand what you can use or buy (organic whenever possible) to ensure that your body will respond well:

Water: Purified. My favorite is Hinckley Springs Mountain Valley, which comes in glass five-gallon (19-liter) containers.

Raw vegetables: Try to eat a rainbow of various colors each day. If organic lettuces come in a bag, these are okay, but fresher and locally grown is even better.

Raw fruit: All are okay, but if you eat a banana, try to eat only half a banana daily. An apple a day helps if you have trouble sleeping.

Blended fresh vegetables or fruit: Okay and good if you have digestive issues. Try to consume them within 15 minutes to preserve enzymes.

Juiced fresh vegetables or fruit: Okay. If you have a twin-gear or a centrifugal juicer, you may store your juice in a glass container in your refrigerator for a couple of days. The enzymes do not suffer as much damage from the heating of a single-gear juicer.

Mushrooms: Raw and cleaned well. Peel the scales from the underside of Portobellos.

Olives: Raw fats found in avocados, olives, coconuts, nuts, and seeds are important in a healthy diet. These fats are antioxidant-rich and contain oils that help the joints, bones, and nerves. Sun-dried olives are the best. Many olives in a jar have been cooked.

Sprouts: Grow your own. It only takes a few days to do so, and the result is an enzyme-rich food that is second to none. Soak alfalfa or other seeds overnight. Drain and rinse them. Allow them to sprout in a glass dish or bowl that is covered lightly. Rinse daily, and when you are content with the sprouts, soak them for a few minutes in vinegar water and drain. Put the covered dish in the refrigerator and use over salads, in romaine tacos, or in smoothies.

Dried sea vegetables: These are iodine and mineral-rich to support the endocrine system. One tablespoon (15 ml) of dulse or kelp daily is very helpful. Sprinkle on salads or in raw soups or patés.

CHAPTER 10

The Green Line and Transitional Diets

The truth is fasting is one of the safest healing methods known to medical science. As a matter of fact, you can live without food for months, but you can kill yourself by overeating in a few weeks.
—DR. PAAVO AIROLA, *HOW TO KEEP SLIM, HEALTHY, AND YOUNG WITH JUICE FASTING*

I have developed a philosophy concerning the American diet that I call the "Green Line" (see Table 10-1). It is like a map that explains where you are in terms of your diet and where you need to be to achieve and maintain vibrant health. Imagine a long line across the page from left to right. At the beginning of the line would be number one, a base of individuals who eat the freshest and best foods available to humans on the planet. These foods consist of fresh, organic, easy-to-digest and -absorb, enzyme-rich, raw fruits and vegetables. At the opposite end of the line, number twenty, are the worst foods that a person could possibly consume. These foods are dead, difficult-to-digest and -absorb, overcooked, synthetic, acidic, processed products. This is the quick stop, rip it out of the bag and eat it diet. This is bagged, boxed, bottled, dead shelf food that is packed with foodless foods, preservatives, sodium, and sugar. You eat foods that place you on this line somewhere. In my experience, the Green Line might look like this (see opposite page) if we consider the number of potential people in each particular category. Unfortunately, there are probably as many people in the one to four categories as the nine to ten.

I created the theory of the Green Line to gain a better, more helpful perspective about where an individual's eating habits are so I could talk to them about what they need to do to try to eat better. This is in no way a judgment,

TABLE 10-1 THE GREEN LINE DIET									
25% POPULATION			MAJORITY 50% POPULATION			25% POPULATION			
1–4			5–8			9–10			
1	2	3	4	5	6	7	8	9	10

MIGHT BE PRIMARY FOODS	MIGHT BE BEVERAGES OF CHOICE
1. Raw vegan fruit & vegetables—100% organic	Water, tea, raw juices (some drink rejeuvelac)
2. High raw vegan (80% raw)— 100% organic fruits and vegetables	Water, tea, raw juices (some drink rejeuvelac)
3. Vegan (50% raw)—vegetables and fruit, organic cooked foods, legumes, grains. No animal products	Water, tea, raw juices, organic coffee
4. Vegetarian (25% raw vegetables)—with eggs, dairy, cooked foods, some processed mostly organic	Water, tea, juices, organic coffee, some alcohol
5. Fish, vegetables (25% raw)—with eggs, pasta, dairy, some processed mostly organic	Water, tea, juices, milk, coffee, alcohol
6. Fish, chicken, dairy, vegetables (25% raw)— processed foods, some organic	Water, tea, juice, soda, coffee, milk, alcohol
7. Red meat (1 time a week), fish, chicken, dairy, some vegetables (10% raw)—processed foods	Water, tea, juice, soda, milk, coffee, alcohol
8. Meats daily, canned fruits and vegetables, processed foods, breads, sugar, and candy	Water, tea, juice, soda, milk, coffee, alcohol
9. Red meat, fast food 4+ times per week, chicken and dairy, pre-packaged foods, breads, candy, sugar, and less than 1 vegetable daily	Sweet tea, coffee, milk, alcohol, soda
10. Mostly red meat, fast food, chips, candy, cheese, breads, sugars, ice cream, no vegetables.	Soda, coffee, milk, alcohol, no water

just a tool for dietary transition. If a person is a ten, they might have a difficult time making a dietary leap all the way back to one. But if they are a five already, the job is easier. Check to see where you fall on the Green Line and ask yourself what changes you might make to move in a positive direction.

I have always found that with the proper incentive, a human being can be quite creative. For example, if a person has a life-threatening disease, she will want to find her way back to one or two in a hurry. Frequently, I find that the most difficult change may actually come from a seven, eight, or nine who has an illusion about her true food reality. Most in that range are eating what, unfortunately, has been labeled the "Standard American Diet," also known as SAD, and do not consider it unusual or unhealthy because most of their peers and the commercials they see on television support their poor eating habits. In most cases, an individual scoring a nine or a ten recognizes that her diet is unwise.

I do not mention the advantages of organic foods, but consider it a must in all cases. Chances are, people eating in the six-to-ten range do not consider organic of importance. While people at all socioeconomic levels eat in the nine-to-ten range, unfortunately, it is often a diet associated with poverty or individuals who do not have the means or the will to shop beyond the convenience mart and the fast-food restaurants.

The Green Line might give you some perspective about how you might change one or two bad habits to put yourself in a greener place on the line. I feel that it reflects better health habits and health and immunity directly.

THE GREEN LINE AND THE GUNAS

The Green Line for Sattvic foods might run from one to three. The Sattvic foods are primarily sweet, fresh, and agreeable. These include leafy green vegetables, other vegetables, fruits, nuts, seeds, whole grains, honey, pure water, and teas.

The Rajasic foods on the Green Line might consist of numbers four through nine. These foods include stimulating and acidic foods, like meat, fish, processed foods, and chocolate. They are said to create restlessness in the mind. Eating too fast or with a disturbed or stressed mind is also considered rajasic. The emotions that accompany raja are frustration, feeling manic or hyper, unsettled, and with a compulsive need to control your environment or others around you just to feel safe.

Tamasic food is considered to be poisonous. This holds position ten on the Green Line. It creates a dullness of the mind and obscures the thinking. It involves overeating the wrong kinds of foods—those that are dead, stale, and overripe. This diet includes alcohol, processed foods and meats, and few or no fresh foods. The emotions that accompany these foods are aggression, hopelessness, and depression.

THE GREEN LINE TRANSITION TO A RAW FOODS DIET

TRANSITION ONE: Adding Fresh Foods and Enzymes to the Diet

If you are a nine or a ten on the Green Line, I would recommend that you follow the following suggestions to move toward a raw diet. Following these will help you on your way to an easier transition. With cooked meals, I always suggest consuming two or three betaine hydrochloric acid (HCl) 350 mg capsules ten minutes before eating, but if you forget, take them later. Hydrochloric acid remains available in the stomach for later digestive processes.

A new patient came into our clinic, and after reviewing his diet of fast food from two nationally famous competing burger companies and his six cans of diet soda daily, I asked him why he ate fast food and soda at every meal. His reply was quick. First, he liked the taste of those big fast-food burgers and fries; second, it was cheap and easy. He was overweight, unhealthy, and unhappy. "Is it worth it?" I asked.

He seemed surprised that I had asked him such a question. No one ever had. "Is what worth it?"

"Is your fast-food diet making your life better or worse? Are you investing your food dollars for health or toward something that robs you of your health?" He'd never thought of food as an investment before. He could wrap his mind around the idea of a bad investment. I spoke to him about how a better diet could make him feel better by allowing enzymes and nutrients in fruits and vegetables to work for him. I challenged him to eat 50 percent raw vegetables and fruit daily and to avoid fast food and soda. At his next appointment, two months later, he'd lost eighteen pounds (8 kg) and was excited because he thought nothing would work for him. He'd had his doubts, but now he was determined.

If you drink soda pop, cut your consumption in half each week and replace it with pure water or herbal tea. By the third week, you should no longer be drinking soda at all. Soda pop may be the number one source of sugar in your diet. To determine how much sugar is in a can of soda, you need to do a little math. A Nutrition Facts panel for a twelve-ounce (340 g) can of soda lists 48 grams of total carbohydrates. Divide 48 by 4 to get 12, the number of teaspoons of sugar in this can. If you drink this, you will be drinking 12 teaspoons (60 ml) of sugar. For larger bottles of soda, you need to multiply the number of teaspoons of sugar for one serving by the number of servings that is indicated on the bottle. Sugar appears on the label as corn syrup, high-fructose corn syrup, sugar, and sucrose. Children should not be drinking soda pop, and its consumption has been linked with type 1 or juvenile onset diabetes.

I have noticed that many people in the eight-to-ten range on the Green Line do not drink enough water to avoid constipation. I tell my patients, "Never let the sun set without a bowel movement. Make it happen with a glass of water and one tablespoon (15 ml) of Epsom salts, repeat every two hours until you have success. Next day, double your plant fiber by eating six cups (1,200 ml) of mixed salad greens."

Diet for Transition One

Every morning

1. Drink one-half fresh-squeezed lemon in 8 ounces (227 g) of warm water or three tablespoons (45 ml) of organic bottled lemon juice in eight ounces (227 g) of warm water. Wait ten minutes before eating.

2. Alternate for 1 week: Raw green smoothie (see recipes) and plain oatmeal with agave nectar, almond milk, and either blueberries or strawberries. No dairy. Eggs are okay in moderation twice a week.

3. Drink 1 cup (200 ml) of organic coffee or green tea. If your cholesterol is high, drink alfalfa tea and take two to three garlic tablets containing about 9 mg allicin daily.

4. Take 4–6 chlorella tablets (or 20–30 grams) daily in the morning.

5. Take two refrigerated probiotic (containing both acidophilus and bifidum) capsules daily, especially if you have taken antibiotics in the past year.

6. Consider a good colon cleansing product, like Blue Heron, or a blend that contains psyllium, Bentonite clay, and senna, triphala, or cascara in a capsule or powder daily.

   As a snack: fruit, celery, carrots, trail mix (no peanuts), raw bar, cacao mix. No candy or chocolate (other than raw cacao.)

Lunch

1. Fish one day, chicken the next. No bread. Only 1 serving per day.

2. Brown rice or brown rice pasta (many brands found in grocery stores).

3. Lentils, black beans, pinto beans, or red beans.

4. Soup with vegetarian broth.

5. Large salad (no iceberg lettuce) if fish or chicken is eaten at dinner.

6. Purified water or a cup (200 ml) of green tea or organic coffee

Dinner

1. Once a week, red meat the size of a deck of cards, or fish or chicken if none is eaten at lunch.

2. If you are not eating fish or chicken, have a large chef's salad with mixed greens, avocado, red pepper (not green), sunflower seeds, and goat, feta, or mozzarella cheese (see recipes for dressing). If you are eating fish or chicken, a smaller salad is recommended, or steamed vegetables like broccoli, cauliflower, green beans, or edamame.

3. Brown rice pasta with one cup (200 ml) frozen or fresh broccoli or spinach plunged into the boiling pasta water in the last two minutes of cooking. Toss with garlic tomato sauce or salad dressing with chopped kalamata olives and goat feta or mozzarella.

4. Veggie burger with gluten-free bun and organic ketchup. Steamed kale or chard with toasted sesame seeds. Lightly boiled small organic potatoes topped with olive oil or toasted sesame oil.

5. Water or chamomile tea.

Snack: To aid with sleep and maintaining blood sugar levels

1. Slices of raw pineapple.

2. Apple slices with walnuts and cinnamon.

3. Blueberry smoothie (see recipes).

TRANSITION TWO: Moving Toward Vegetarian and Raw Foods

If you are a seven or eight on the Green Line, you may follow the following suggestions in progressing toward a vegetarian raw diet. If you followed Transition One for two weeks to a month, you are ready to move on to Transition Two. This is a healthy vegetarian diet. You may choose to sustain Transition Two after you have completed my three-month 4-3-2-1 raw diet. Once you are restored to health, you might decide that you want to add in some animal protein. In that case, I would consider red meat only once a week. The serving amount of animal protein should not exceed the size of a deck of cards, and poultry or fish no more than three times a week—a total of both. Please keep in mind that a greens-rich, alkaline vegetarian diet (daily servings of six vegetables, two fruits, one starch, one vegetable protein like lentils or beans) is the healthiest diet on the planet. Avoiding chocolate or candy may be challenging for you, so I suggest you find a substitute like raw cacao with dates and nuts processed into raw refrigerator cookies, or just a date (with the seed removed) stuffed with a Brazil nut. If you are reading this book, I know you are motivated enough to find a replacement for that addictive food, which is a health stealer.

Breakfast, Lunch, or Dinner: Eat a wide variety of vegetables and fruits daily

1. Eat 1 very large (6 cups [1,200 ml]) salad daily with crunchy vegetables and nuts. Top with your choice of raw dressings. Eat six servings of vegetables daily, mostly raw. Eighty percent of your diet should be raw organic.

2. Eat soaked nuts, 6 tablespoons (90 ml) daily for snacks or on salads.

3. Twice weekly eat sprouts, especially alfalfa, quinoa, and lentils.

4. Eat 2 different types of fruit daily; only one-half banana daily.

5. Eat 1 green smoothie daily with green or red apple or pear.

6. You may eat one cooked meal daily, but when you do, I would consider taking betaine hydrochloric acid (HCl), especially when consuming cooked beans like black beans, red beans, pinto beans, or lentils.

7. Eat a cup or two of miso soup, especially in the colder months. Add crushed garlic, seaweed, sprouted grains, chopped spinach, or broccoli.

8. Eat one-half avocado three to four times a week.

9. Allowable additions: 1 tablespoon (15 ml) dulse or kelp to raw soups or salads, 1 tablespoon (15 ml) cinnamon on fruit, raw organic hemp seed for salads or soups as well as olives, avocado, celery, onion, garlic, ground flax or sesame seeds.

10. No cow dairy, like cheese, butter, milk, cream. No eggs. No sugar or bread unless it is gluten-free and in moderation, not to exceed four slices weekly. Top with raw almond butter, raw veggies to make a salad sandwich—not tuna or chicken. Toasted top with sesame oil.

11. Consider drinking at least six to eight 10-ounce (283 g) glasses of purified water daily (for 120- to 160-pound [54–73 kg] adults). Also beneficial are green or herbal teas and no more than 2 cups (400 ml) of organic coffee daily. If you like cream in your coffee, transition to coconut milk or make your own calcium-rich almond or sesame milk with just a blender, water, and almond or sesame seeds (see recipes). If you like sugar in your coffee, transition to agave nectar or raw honey.

TRANSITION THREE: Raw Smoothies or Juicing

You might decide that juice fasting or drinking raw smoothies is an easier way for you to transition to a raw diet, or you might consider it as a way to detoxify on a regular basis. If you have a health concern, please refer to my information about healing diseases with raw fruits and vegetables. You may also decide that you would like to do weekend juicing or smoothies. Some people prefer smoothies to juicing because it involves easier cleanup and less costly investment in machinery. Good juicers are a premium, but worth every penny. We have owned many different styles and prefer the centrifugal type for its easy cleanup and preservation of enzymes. We usually make two days' worth of juice at a time and drink raw juice every morning for breakfast. It takes us about twenty minutes, or at the most, half an hour with cleanup. That means about ten to twenty minutes each morning to prepare a great breakfast. When we travel, we always take our Vita Mix and prepare smoothies for breakfast. Nothing jumpstarts your day like those precious enzymes. You have to find a convenient way to make enzymes part of your healthier lifestyle. Below are some recipes for the three-day smoothie or juice "fast." Juice-fasting is a means of detoxifying that also allows you to lose about ten pounds (4.5 kg) a week. We call it fasting even though it is more than water because it is a fluid-based healing diet. Remember to review those other fruits or vegetables that might help you create your own weekend juice fast. I recommend ten ounces (283 g) of juice for each "meal."

CHAPTER 11

Raw Juice-Fasting and Fasting with Smoothies

Often in this technological age where computers diagnose diseases and perform surgery, we tend to minimize natural therapies. It seems incredible that the simple act of drinking raw juices could turn around severe diseases, however I have seen it work in otherwise hopeless cases.

—Dr. Sandra Cabot, *Raw Juices Can Save Your Life,* www.liverdoctor.com

WEEKEND JUICE OR SMOOTHIE FAST

Note: Use organic produce whenever possible or substitute organic frozen fruits or vegetables when fresh is not available. Our favorite is locally grown produce, but ensure that it is chemical and pesticide free before you purchase it.

SHOPPING LIST: Add or subtract according to your health needs

Note: If you have greens in your refrigerator, please use those in the recipes first.

Produce

Vegetables

1 large head romaine or package of 3 romaine hearts

1 bundle of spinach or 1 box organic baby spinach

1 bunch cilantro (optional)

1 small bunch kale (lacinato, darkest green)

1 bunch organic celery

1 large or two small beets with tops

1 small bunch broccoli

8 carrots

2 or 3 cucumbers

Fruit

1 fresh pineapple

4 Granny Smith apples

2 Asian or 3 Bartlett or Bosc pears

1 small ginger root

2 avocados

1 orange

2 lemons or bottled 16-ounce (0.5 kg) organic lemon juice (not raw)

1 banana

1 small bunch of purple seedless grapes or 1 small package strawberries

Optional: 1 kiwi, 1 peach, 2 dates

Other Additions

1 package sesame seeds or jar of tahini

1 package raw flax seeds or refrigerated flax oil; highest lignan is best

1 package short-grain, or Wehani or Lundberg Farms rice (optional)

1 jar raw almond butter

1 jar or 4 tablespoons (60 ml) fresh cinnamon

Optional: Brewer's yeast, gluten free vanilla. Wheatgrass juice. Teas: chamomile, Pau D'arco, nettle.

Optional: valerian, goldenseal, dandelion leaf (as a natural diuretic with beneficial potassium), chlorella powder, spirulina

Smoothies

Smoothies and juice are both healthy and beneficial to achieve or maintain wellness. They are both made from organic fruits and vegetables. The primary difference between the two is fiber. When you juice, the fiber or pulp is separated from the liquid. With smoothies, the fiber is an integral part of what you drink. I would not encourage keeping smoothies for more than a half a day, but juice that has been processed through a twin-gear or centrifugal juicer can be kept for up to three days. Single-gear juicers tend to heat the enzymes and kill them, so your window of opportunity for storage is about twenty minutes. Each day you store your juice in the refrigerator, you lose some of the enzymes. Another difference is that with smoothies, you might need to add some type of liquid, like purified water or the milks and teas listed below. When juice fasting is indicated, no fiber is allowed in the drink because it activates the digestive processes and creates feelings of hunger. For that reason, when you're juice-fasting, straining the juice is an important step.

Another important step in drinking smoothies or juice is to swish the fluid in your mouth for a few seconds to release saliva into the juice before swallowing. This is the first step in digestion, and it's vital for a comfortable stomach and easier breakdown of juice.

In all cases, there are certain food contraindications for juicing and smoothies, as noted below:

1. If you are taking a prescription heart medication, avoid grapefruit.

2. If you have high blood pressure, avoid ginger or licorice tea.

3. If you are on a juice fast, I suggest that you avoid vitamin tablets or capsules. Powders or liquid nutrients may be added. If you are taking a prescription medication, it is important that you continue doing so and check with your physician about fasting.

4. If you are juicing citrus, it is best to peel or use only half the skin of the organic fruit only.

5. The seeds of apples should be removed before juicing; they contain trace amounts of cyanide. Some people do not bother.

6. Avoid goitrogens if they are contraindicated with your thyroid disorder. These are members of the cabbage family that can block the usefulness of iodine to your body.

7. If you have cancer, avoid all carrots, citrus, and fruits in general; the exception one-half Granny Smith apple used for juicing.

RECIPES FOR MILKS AND TEAS TO ADD TO SMOOTHIES

RAW RICE MILK

Raw rice milk can be very bitter. It is the macrobiotic remedy for cancer, especially bone cancer. Because rice is bitter, consider sprouting instead. Organic short- or medium-grain rice is preferable for making raw rice milk.

Directions for Sprouting Rice Grains

Rinse 1 cup (200 ml) of rice and soak it for ten minutes in vinegar water. Rinse it again and put it in a glass or a stainless-steel bowl and cover it with 2 cups (400 ml) purified water to leave overnight. Drain and rinse it the next morning. You may use this in rice milk then or allow it to sprout for one more day in the same container with no water. At this point you could eat the chewy rice as a base for mushrooms, shredded carrots, red peppers (stir, not fried). Rinse before using.

Ingredients for Raw Rice Milk

1 cup (200 ml) sprouted raw rice grains

4 cups (800 ml) purified water

Directions for Raw Rice Milk

Blend until grains are liquefied. Strain through a fine-wire strainer (the easier way) or cheesecloth. Wring the cheesecloth to remove all fluids.

Save the pulp and blend with 1 tablespoon (15 ml) of raw miso as a poultice or compress for inflamed tissue anywhere on the body. Leave directly on the skin for half an hour. Refrigerate and reuse or discard in a compost heap.

EASIEST RAW SESAME MILK

Ingredients

1 cup (200 ml) of unhulled sesame seeds
rinsed in vinegar water and soaked overnight

3 cups (600 ml) of purified water

Variations: 1 teaspoon (5 ml) vanilla, $1/2$ teaspoon (3 ml) cinnamon,
1 teaspoon (5 ml) agave

Directions

Blend all ingredients until seeds are liquefied. Strain through a fine-wire mesh or cheesecloth. Compost the remains or use 1 tablespoon (15 ml) daily in a smoothie.

EASIEST EVER SESAME MILK

Put $1/4$ cup (50 ml) raw sesame butter in 3 cups (600 ml) purified water. Blend. Store this in a quart jar in the refrigerator. In smoothies, it is easier to just put 2 tablespoons (30 ml) of sesame tahini (or any kind of nut butter except peanuts, which are legumes, not nuts) into the blender with 1 cup (200 ml) of water and the remaining raw ingredients. Keep in mind that tahini is generally not found on grocery shelves, but it is nutrient-rich. Add $1/2$ teaspoon (3 ml) vanilla or cinnamon, if desired.

EASIEST EVER ALMOND MILK

Put $1/4$ cup (50 ml) raw almond butter in 3 cups (600 ml) purified water. Blend. In smoothies, it is easier to just put 2 tablespoons (30 ml) of almond butter (or any kind of nut butter, except peanut butter) into the blender with 1 cup (200 ml) of water and the rest of the raw ingredients.

POTASSIUM TEA

Scrub and soak in vinegar water 8 medium potatoes. Peel the potatoes, leaving the skin thick, and boil the skins in a quart (1 liter) of water for 10 minutes. Let it steep for another 10 minutes and strain. Drink a warm cup daily, especially at night during juice-fasting. *Optional:* Boil with 6 cloves of garlic and or a cup (200 ml) of parsley.

YOUNG COCONUT MILK

Using extreme caution, cut off the tops of four young coconuts by shaving back the white layer at the top until about three inches is exposed, and then strike it near the lower band that was peeled with a large knife or meat cleaver. Seek more directions online, if needed. Pop it off and then pour the contents into a blender or Vita Mix. Scrape out the "pudding." Blend all until smooth, then store in a glass jar and refrigerate. Compost the coconut shells. This is delicious in smoothies.

FLAXSEED TEA

Put 1 tablespoon (15 ml) of organic, ground (not whole) flax seeds into 2 1/2 cups (500 ml) of purified water. Bring to a boil, then simmer for 5 minutes. Turn off the heat and steep ten minutes. Strain out the seeds and sip the tea slowly. I suggest this method rather than a tea ball or cup strainer because the mucus of the flax gets in the way of straining and absorption. This tea is especially nurturing for the gallbladder and most useful during a gallbladder attack.

CINNAMON FLAXSEED TEA

Ingredients

4 tablespoons (60 ml) ground, organic flax seed

2 cups (400 ml) boiling water

1/2 teaspoon (3 ml) ground cinnamon

Variation: 1/2 teaspoon (3 ml) agave nectar

Directions

Put ground flax and cinnamon into a teapot or cup. Pour the boiling water over it and allow it to steep ten minutes. Strain and drink. This is especially helpful as a mild bowel stimulant.

GREEN TEAS

Green tea and certain mushrooms contain L-theanine, which produces a calming effect on the body. My favorite type of green tea is called Genmai, which contains a mixture, usually in equal parts, of green tea and roasted brown rice. It is called the "snap, crackle, and pop" of green teas. It was once a peasant's drink to extend the tea, but is now considered quite chic. High-quality green tea is very soothing, and the caffeine is not as strong as in coffee. While there has been a rebirth of hot water tea decaffeination, this ancient method does not work well with all kinds of green teas. If you are concerned about caffeine, pour a third of a cup of hot water over the tea leaves, steep for about a minute, and then pour out the liquid that contains most of the caffeine. Add the appropriate amount of hot water to the damp leaves, and steep this second round of tea about a minute and a half. Many fine tea connoisseurs would consider this a waste of the best part of the tea.

TABLE 11.1   NUTRIENT VALUES PRESENT IN DR. MITCHELL'S RAW GREEN JUICE OR SMOOTHIE

NUTRIENT	DAILY VALUES	IN 10 OUNCES (284 G) GREEN SMOOTHIE
Vitamin A	5,000 IU	600–6,000 IU
Vitamin C	60 mg (500 x 2)	200 mg
Calcium	1,000 mg	500 mg
Iron	18 mg	55 mg
Vitamin D	400 IU (2,000 D_3)	sunlight/liquid drops
Vitamin E	30 IU (300 IU)	60 IU
Vitamin K	80 mcg	150 mcg
Thiamine	1.5 mg	0.5 mg
Riboflavin (B_2)	1.7 mg	1 mg
Niacin	20 mg	15 mg
Vitamin B_6	2.0 (20 mg)	2.25 mg
Folic acid B_9/Folate	400 mcg	83 mcg

B$_{12}$	6.0 mcg	liquid drops
Biotin	300 mcg	0.06 mg
Pantothentic acid	10 –15 mg	—
Phosphorus	1,000 mg	—
Potassium	—	600–1,500 mg
Iodine	150 mcg	(Add kelp)
Magnesium	400 mg or more	250–600mg
Zinc	15–50 mg	35 mg
Copper	2.0 mg	—
Manganese	2.0	—

One of the fantastic side effects of green smoothies is that they detoxify inorganic xenotoxins and metals. As you can see in Table 11-1, there are some nutrients not listed in the green smoothie due to lack of these in depleted soils. Since that is the case, for those who are juice-fasting I suggest supplementing with professional liquid vitamin sources for longer than seven days. In Ayurveda, water is left overnight in small copper cups to drink the next morning as a way to supplement the body's need for copper. It is a cofactor offered with DHEA that European research has found useful in repairing the myelin sheath in patients suffering from multiple sclerosis.

JUICE OR SMOOTHIE:
GENERAL NUTRITION INFORMATION

You may wish to check the general nutritional content in each smoothie recipe per vegetables added in order to receive the amounts of specific nutrition that you desire.

Romaine lettuce (the darker the lettuce, the more nutrient content): Protein, vitamins A and C, thiamine, riboflavin, B$_6$, niacin, folic acid, potassium, calcium, magnesium, sodium, phosphorus, iron.

Ginger: Ginger is used primarily as a soother for the gastrointestinal system. It is warming for the system because juices tend to cause "cool dampness."

Ginger, like fennel, relieves intestinal gas, it acts as an anti-inflammatory, and it relaxes the intestinal tract for better digestion.

Broccoli and kale: Protein, vitamins A and C, thiamine, riboflavin, B_6, niacin, folic acid, potassium, calcium, magnesium, sodium, phosphorus, and iron.

Cucumber: Protein, vitamins A and C, thiamine, riboflavin, niacin, B_6, folic acid, magnesium, sodium, phosphorus, potassium, calcium, iron.

Celery: Protein, vitamins A and C, thiamine, riboflavin, B_6, niacin, folic acid, potassium, calcium, magnesium, sodium, phosphorus, iron.

Apple and pear: Protein, vitamins A and C, thiamine, riboflavin, niacin, folic acid, potassium, calcium, magnesium, sodium, phosphorus, iron (pear helps to relieve constipation).

Carrots: Vitamins A and C, thiamine, B_6, niacin, folic acid, protein, potassium, magnesium, phosphorus, sodium, iron, calcium.

Beets (tops are considered greens and have more nutritional value than the root): Protein, vitamins A and C, thiamine, riboflavin, B_6, niacin, folic acid, potassium, calcium, magnesium, sodium, phosphorus, and iron.

Garlic: Garlic contains sulfur compounds that have many therapeutic effects. Garlic has proven beneficial in lowering blood sugar and protecting against cancer. It has antifungal, antibacterial, and anti-parasitic properties, and it enhances the immune system and detoxifies the body of heavy metals. I might suggest three cloves of raw garlic daily in smoothies or juice when you are not going out in public. We juice garlic at the very end of the juicing process and make two equal batches of juice—one with the juiced garlic for later in the day, and one without for fresher breath during the day.

B_{12}: Consider adding B_{12} drops daily to juice or smoothies if you're engaged in extended fasting.

THE WEEKEND SMOOTHIE DETOX PLAN

Friday Evening

JUICE OR SMOOTHIE: GREEN MOVER

Ingredients

1 Asian or organic Bartlett pear

4 ounces (113 g) of spinach (2 cups [400 ml])

3 stalks of celery

1 carrot

1 cucumber

1 Granny Smith apple

2 dates or 1 prune

If you're making a smoothie: 2 cups (400 ml) water

Directions

For Smoothie: Cut apples and pear into 4 sections and remove seeds. Place water in blender and add all ingredients except greens. Blend until smooth and add in greens and finally the dates or prune. Blend until creamy. Pour into glasses.

For Juice: Cut fruit into 4 sections and remove the seeds. Vegetables and fruit need to be sliced thin enough to fit into the feeding tube of the juicer. Juice all ingredients; water is not needed. Compost the plant waste—it now has little nutritional value. Pour the juice and drink.

Try to save 6 ounces (170 g) of this smoothie for an 8:00 a.m. snack.

Before bed: 1 cup chamomile tea or potassium tea

Saturday Morning

$1/_2$ lemon squeezed into 8 ounces (227 g) of warm water drink at least 15 minutes before juice

Flaxseed tea

10–12 ounces (284–340 g) water

R & S (RISE N' SHINE) JUICE

Ingredients

1 orange

2 cups (400 ml) raw pineapple

1 Granny Smith apple

$\frac{1}{2}$ Bartlett pear

$\frac{1}{2}$ peach

1 cup of pre-washed spinach greens

2 cups (400 ml) water

Variations: If you're making a smoothie,
blend 1 teaspoon (5 ml) Brewer's yeast
and 1 tablespoon (15 ml) ground sesame or flax seeds

Directions

For Smoothie: Cut apples, peach, and orange into 4 sections and remove seeds. It is not necessary to peel anything but the pineapple. Chop pineapple into large chunks. Place water in blender and add all ingredients except greens. Blend until smooth and add in greens and any ingredients for the variation you'd like to use. Blend until creamy. Pour into glasses and enjoy.

For Juice: Cut fruit into 4 sections and remove the seeds. Peel and slice pineapple into strips. Vegetables and fruit need to be sliced thin enough to fit into the feeding tube of the juicer. Juice all ingredients, water is not needed. Compost the discarded plant waste, it now has little nutritional value. Pour the juice and drink.

Midmorning tea: Alfalfa (for high cholesterol, or colon or kidney issues) or nettle tea (for iron deficiency or anemia), strained

Saturday Lunch

RED SNAPPER

Ingredients

2 cups (400 ml) water

2 carrots

1 small beet, plus top

8 romaine leaves

1 apple

broccoli ($\frac{1}{8}$ cup [25 ml])

Directions

For Smoothie: Blend 1 avocado and 1 tablespoon (15 ml) cinnamon.

For Juice: Add 1 tablespoon (15 ml) flax oil and 1 tablespoon (15 ml) cinnamon.

Variation: Add ginger juiced or peeled and sliced into blender (if you don't have high blood pressure).

Midafternoon tea: Pau D'Arco (yeast binder), goldenseal (for colitis or yeast issues), or green tea

Saturday Dinner

ROMANCING THE KALE

Ingredients

4 leaves kale

4 leaves romaine

2 celery stalks

$\frac{1}{2}$ cucumber

1 cup (200 ml) strawberries or grapes

Directions

For Smoothie: Mix all ingredients with 1 tablespoon (15 ml) Brewer's yeast or almond butter.

For Juice: Mix all ingredients and stir in 1 teaspoon (5 ml) chlorella and 2 cups (400 ml) water.

8:00 p.m.: You may have 4 ounces (113 g) of any juice leftovers.

Evening tea: Chamomile or catnip or valerian.

Later: 10 ounces (284 g) water or potassium tea

Sunday Breakfast

PARADISE CALLS

$^1/_2$ lemon squeezed into 8 ounces (227 g) of warm water drink at least 15 minutes before juice.

Ingredients

1 peeled mango

1 avocado

2 cups spinach

1 peeled kiwi

2 stalks celery

1 cup (200 ml) strawberries or purple grapes

Directions

For Smoothie: Mix all ingredients and blend in $^1/_2$ banana and 2 tablespoons (30 ml) almond butter and 2 cups (400 ml) water.

For Juice: Add a slice of ginger, plus 10 ounces (284 g) water to the smoothie. You may save 4 ounces (113 g) of juice for a midafternoon snack.

Tea: Pau D' Arco, alfalfa, green tea, ground flaxseed tea, or nettle tea.

Sunday Lunch

DR. MITCHELL'S MODIFIED JUICE RECIPE

Ingredients

4 leaves of romaine or 1 cup (200 ml) spinach

3 kale leaves

1 Granny Smith apple

1 small beet with green tops

3 celery stalks

1–2 carrots (contraindicated for cancer patients)

Variations: $1/2$ inch (13 mm) slice of raw ginger (optional; not for those with high blood pressure)

1 raw garlic clove (optional)

1 cup of purified water or sesame or almond milk

Directions

For Smoothie: Remove seeds in fruit and quarter. Blend all ingredients and add 2 tablespoons (30 ml) nut butters with 1 cup (200 ml) water.

For Juice: Mix all ingredients and stir in sesame or almond milk. Water is not needed.

You may save 4 ounces (113 g) for an after-dinner snack. Or as an option, see the recipe for the Dinosaur and the Pink Lady.

Tea: Pau D'Arco, alfalfa, dandelion, or nettle

THE DINOSAUR AND THE PINK LADY

Ingredients

1 bunch of dinosaur kale

3–5 carrots with 2 tops (tops are bitter)

3–4 stalks of celery

1½ Bosc or Bartlett pear and or 1½ Pink Lady apple

Variation: If you're making a smoothie, add 1 tablespoon (15 ml) cinnamon and 1 cup (200 ml) almond milk.

Directions

Remove seeds from fruit and blend or juice all ingredients. No water is needed when juicing.

Sunday Dinner: Blend or Juice Whatever's Left

Ingredients

Any beets or leafy salad greens that are left from the weekend

2 leaves of kale

3 small pieces of broccoli

½ cucumber

1 carrot

1–2 stalks of celery

1 slice ginger

Apple or pear or ½ of each

Grapes or strawberries (½–1 cup [100–200 ml])

Directions

For Juice: Add 1 tablespoon (15 ml) flax oil.

Variation: Smoothie: Add 1 tablespoon (15 ml) cinnamon and ground flax seeds.

Tea: Chamomile later *or* 1 cup (200 ml) potassium tea

Or, as an option, see the recipe for Crocodile Stomach below for a stomach that is grumpy or is developing ulcers.

CROCODILE STOMACH

Ingredients

$1/2$ head of red or green cabbage

3 stalks of celery

3 carrots (plus tops)

$1/2$ cup (100 ml) cilantro or parsley

1 cup (200 ml) water

Directions

Wash all produce in vinegar water. Cut cabbage into three-inch chunks. Blend all ingredients. For juicing, no water is needed.

Variation: Add $1/2$ Granny Smith apple, seeds removed.

Optional Sunday dinner addition:

GRAPEFRUIT N' GREENS

Ingredients

2 pink grapefruit

1 lime, peeled

1 apple, cored

Kale leaves, whole

1 cup of purified water

Directions

Remove seeds from fruits. Blend all ingredients. For juicer: no water is needed.

Drink 10 ounces (284 g) of water twice a day.

8:00 p.m.: Juice or smoothie left over from lunch.

Monday Morning

$1/2$ lemon squeezed into 8 ounces (227 g) of warm water drink at least 15 minutes before breakfast. (I do not recommend extended use of lemon juice water as a protocol.)

FLAXSEED TEA (OPTIONAL) OR GREEN TEA

If possible, try a lighter breakfast of mixed fruit, avocado, or an apple with a light coating of almond butter. Break your fast with more alkaline fruits.

As you move into lunch and dinner, remember to start with apple slices, and then later move toward leafy raw greens. Avoid cooked foods for several days.

Other Juice and Smoothie Recipes to Choose from

GREEN PH MONSTER

Ingredients

6 stalks celery

2 Granny Smith apples

2 cups (400 ml) spinach

1 cup (200 ml) parsley or cilantro

Slice of ginger root, $1/2$ inch (13 mm) thick

$1/4$ lime

1 cup (200 ml) purified water

Directions

Remove seeds from apples. Peel lime. Peeling ginger is optional. Blend or juice all ingredients.

TUMMY WARMER

Ingredients

2 lemons

1 inch (2.5 cm) ginger root

4 leaves of kale, Swiss chard, spinach, or romaine

1 cucumber

2 stalks celery

1 cup purified water, optional

Directions

Peel lemons and remove seeds. Blend all ingredients for smoothie. Water is not necessary when juicing the above.

Variation: Add 1–2 peeled oranges to the Tummy Warmer.

GREEN CUCUMBER CATERPILLAR

Ingredients

1–2 cucumbers

6 stalks of celery

1 cup (200 ml) parsley

1/2 cup of purified water

Directions

Blend all ingredients for a smoothie. Water is not necessary for juicing.

Variations: Add a bit of dill or ginger. You may also add peppermint tea while blending a smoothie or stir into juice later.

OCEAN DREAMS

Note: You may use frozen organic produce if fresh organic is not available.

Ingredients

2 cups (400 ml) pineapple

2 oranges or 1 cup (200 ml) orange juice

2 cups (400 ml) mango

1 teaspoon (5 ml) chlorella, wheatgrass, or spirulina (added last)

Directions

Peel oranges and pineapple and cut into bite-sized pieces. Blend or juice all ingredients.

Variation: Optional for smoothies: Add the flesh of 1 avocado. May blend in the chlorella, spirulina, or wheatgrass.

RABBIT'S SPRING GARDEN

Ingredients

2 red radishes

3 carrots and tops

1 cup (200 ml) spinach

$\frac{1}{2}$ cucumber

2 stalks celery

1 small apple

$\frac{1}{2}$ red bell pepper

1 chard leaf

1 cup of purified water

Small piece ginger (optional)

Directions

Remove seeds from apple and bell pepper. Blend all ingredients for smoothie. Water is not necessary for juice.

Variations: If you're making a smoothie, use 1 cup (200 ml) almond, wheatgrass juice, water, or sesame milk.

MIGRAINE NO MORE

This is a refreshing drink, good for digestion and migraines. A bit too pulpy for smoothies, but you might want to give it a try. Ground fennel seed tea is great for gastric disruptions and the gas often created by diverticulitis.

Ingredients

1 raw fennel bulb and greens

1 small beet and tops

2 Granny Smith apples

1 stalk celery

Directions

Because fennel is so fibrous, it is best to use a juicer for this recipe. Remove seeds from apples, chop beet, apples, fennel, and celery into smaller pieces to fit in feeding tube. Juice.

YAM IT UP

Great if you need beta-carotene or extra antioxidants. Cube the yam if you are making a smoothie; use sage tea for an interesting herbal twist or purified water.

Ingredients

1 yam or sweet potato, peeled

2 small Bosc or Bartlett pears

2 pink grapefruit, peeled

2 carrots

1 cup (200 ml) spinach (optional)

1 leaf chard (optional)

1 cup of purified water

Directions

For Smoothie: Cut pears, sweet potato, and grapefruit into four sections and remove seeds. Place water in blender and add all ingredients except greens. Blend until smooth and add in greens. Blend until creamy. Pour into glasses.

For Juice: Cut fruit and sweet potato into four sections and remove the seeds. Vegetables and fruit need to be sliced thin enough to fit into the feeding tube of the juicer. Juice all ingredients, water is not needed. Compost the plant waste, it now has little nutritional value. Pour the juice and drink.

BEET 'N' YAM

Ingredients

1 yam or sweet potato (peeled)

1 beet plus tops

1 lemon, seeded (use juice of lemon only for smoothie)

2 stalks celery

1 piece of raw ginger, about $1/4$ inch (6mm) thick

1 slice sweet onion, peeled

1 cup purified water

Directions

Cube the yam and beet, then add the squeezed lemon juice and $1/2$ cup (100 ml) cold purified water for the smoothie. If you're juicing, you can use $1/2$ of the organic lemon rind scrubbed with vinegar and feed into tube. No water is needed for juicing.

YAM 'N' MELON

A nice refreshing drink if you want a sweeter treat.

Ingredients

Flesh of 1 ripe cantaloupe

1 yam peeled (cubed for smoothies)

3 Bosc pears

1 cup (200 ml) spinach or romaine

1 cup of purified water

Directions

Blend or juice all ingredients. Add 1 cup (200 ml) water for smoothies.

SUMMER SPECIAL

Ingredients

1 cup (200 ml) pineapple, peeled

1 lemon (use the juice only for smoothies)

4 cups (800 ml) watermelon, seeded

3 oranges (juice only for smoothies)

Directions

Blend all ingredients for smoothies; no water needed. For juice, you may choose to juice even scrubbed rind pieces and seeds of the organic watermelon.

RAW JUICE FAST FOR THREE OR SEVEN DAYS

It is best to consult your naturopath or natural health care provider before commencing a seven-day juice fast so all your individual health needs are being addressed during the fast. But make no mistake: I have found that a raw juice fast can reverse many diseases, even life-threatening ones, and firmly set your mind in a healing direction. I have found that it is quite common for individuals to lose ten pounds (4.5 kg) during a week-long juice fast. If weight loss is a goal, I encourage a one-week juice fast every month until your body reaches its optimal weight. When you no longer lose weight fasting every month and remaining on a daily 80 percent raw diet, chances are you have reached homeostasis, or where your body operates at its best.

After one or two days, if you are straining your juice sufficiently, such as with a fine-wire mesh strainer, your cravings and feelings of hunger should disappear. It is important for you to reach a proper alkaline pH and engage most of the colors of the rainbow (at once or spread out in the course of the day) to ensure that you are obtaining all the vital nutrients you need. If this is your first juice fast, you have to take it easy. A short nap during the day is encouraged, and you should not be very active at all during your fast or you will break out in a sweat and might even feel faint or experience a sudden drop in energy. I also encourage you to fast with a coach or a partner. If you find a particular juice recipe tasty, then keep it in your repertoire. If not, do not force yourself to drink something too sweet. It never ends well with too much citrus on a protracted raw juice fast. Make sure that you have plenty of raw juice, teas, and organic potatoes for your potassium tea before you start. I also like Emergen-C Lite with MSM (methyl sulfonyl methane, plant-based) twice a day. Do not get stuck without raw juice or tea to nourish your body. Planning is crucial to this fast. It is important to drink several glasses of purified—not distilled—water during your fast to prevent dehydration. You may drink juice, tea, or water whenever you have hunger cravings.

I list below the most alkaline recipes I would use during a juice fast. My juice detox is one that we always use exclusively during our seven-day juice fasts. Some people like to mix up their recipes; other people like to keep it simple by sticking with just one recipe juice that makes shopping easier. No nut milks should be added to juices.

The alkaline juice recipe that I developed for a local organic distributor in the Chicago area is as follows:

DR. MITCHELL'S RAW JUICE DETOX

6 leaves of romaine or 1 cup (200 ml) spinach

3 leaves of collards or kale

3 dandelion leaves

1 Granny Smith or Fuji apple or 1 pear

1 small beet with green tops

3 celery stalks

1 or 2 carrots (contraindicated for cancer patients)

4 inches (10 cm) burdock root (Gabo)

$\frac{1}{2}$-inch (13 mm) slice of raw ginger
(optional; not for those with high blood pressure)

1 raw garlic clove (optional, not recommended
if you are going to be around people)

1 cup of water, wheatgrass, or nettle tea

Directions

For Smoothie: Cut apple or pear into 4 sections and remove seeds. Place water in blender and add all ingredients except greens. Blend until smooth and add in greens. Blend until creamy. Pour into glasses.

For Juice: Cut fruit into four sections and remove the seeds. Vegetables and fruit need to be sliced thin enough to fit into the feeding tube of the juicer. Juice all ingredients; water is not needed. Compost the plant waste, it now has little nutritional value. Pour the juice and drink.

If you leave out the added water, teas, or other fluids, other smoothie recipes can be used as juice recipes for the juice fasting, including the following:

Dr. Mitchell's Raw Juice Detox
or Dr. Mitchell's Modified Juice Recipe

Kale and Delicious

Red Snapper

Green Mover (no dates or prunes)

Crocodile Stomach

The Dinosaur and the Pink Lady

Rabbit's Spring Garden

Remember to add a teaspoon (5 ml) or more of iodine-rich, soaked and strained kelp, nori, dulse water, or radishes to the recipes listed above if you need to shore up your thyroid. Also see list of contraindications specified earlier, and avoid sweeteners unless you use stevia. While it is definitely recommended that you avoid caffeine during a juice fast, if refraining from caffeine keeps you from fasting, one cup (200 ml) of organic coffee might be a viable compromise to your daily routine.

Several good teas include Pau D'Arco, if you are prone to yeast issues. Shave grass, oat straw, corn silk, marshmallow, gravel root, or uva ursi herbal teas are beneficial if your kidneys need support.

I suggest that you start your juice-fasting at the evening meal, and if you have a juicer that does not destroy enzymes (like a centrifugal or twin-gear juicer), you can make enough juice for the next day as well. Store it in a glass container in the refrigerator. The goal is to make juicing and cleanup an easier experience than you would expect. I suggest that you break your fast slowly with apple slices or a light salad. Eating a large or cooked meal after a fast should be avoided. I suggest that you continue eating lots of alkaline greens in the following days.

CHAPTER 12

The Importance of Organic Raw Juice and Smoothies

Fasting is the oldest therapeutic method known to man.
Throughout the long medical history, fasting has been regarded as
one of the most dependable curative and rejuvenative measures.
Hippocrates, "the Father of Medicine," prescribed it. So did Galen,
Paracelsus, and all the other great physicians. Paracelsus called
fasting the "greatest remedy; the physician within."

—DR. PAAVO AIROLA, *JUICE FASTING*

I have never found a quicker way to reduce swelling and reverse disease processes than through the use of raw, strained, juice fasting. When there is an inflammation in the stomach or intestines, areas that are relatively nerve-free, we get what is called "referred pain." This referred pain often is felt in the flank, back, or shoulders. Strained, raw juice is much easier to ingest and absorb that eating a big bowl of fibrous raw fruits and vegetables. In other words, while I am an advocate of a raw diet, there are specific times when it is useful or essential to juice-fast. It is safe and effective, but I feel you must study the process and find a way to ease your mind when it comes to its obsession with cooked food.

An intern who studied with me learned the power of raw foods for healing from our classes and suggested a raw juice fast for a patient who had terminal lung cancer. When you have been given a death sentence, you tend to be more open to helpful suggestions. After three months of raw juicing, the lung cancer was gone; after six months, the patient was out of bed, off oxygen, and resuming a relatively normal life. This patient is considered cured.

128

I know of other doctors who have used raw juicing for the young and old as a means to fight cancer, skin and autoimmune diseases, and gallbladder, pancreas, and liver problems. Chronic diseases seem to melt away with weight as you embrace a raw juice fast. It is the fastest way that I know to provide your body with the nutrients that it needs to heal. Look at a huge bowl of leafy and cruciferous raw vegetables and throw an apple and a small piece of ginger on top of it. When you juice that bowl, chances are that you will end up with maybe twenty ounces (567 g) of juice. When you drink that, it is like receiving a blood plasma transfusion. The body responds quickly to the vitamin-rich liquid. If you find the taste too strong, you can dilute the juice with purified water. If you are diabetic or have cancer, it is generally suggested that you avoid fruits in your juice and use only vegetables.

During raw juicing, you can add supportive nutritional powders dissolved in either purified water or directly in the juice itself. These might include magnesium-calcium powder in a ratio of approximately 1:2 (magnesium 450 mg, calcium 900–1,000 mg). You could add additional vitamin C powder (or a fructose-free C with other vitamins included)—about 1,000 to 2,000 mg daily. There are powdered B supplements, or you could use a capsule that you open and add to the juice. L-glutamine or bromelain powder may help reduce the inflammatory process when taken away from the juice itself and used as a powder added to water. If you add powdered bromelain, which is a pineapple extract, to your juice it becomes a digestive. Raw pineapple fruit is a great medicinal agent that reduces inflammation, aids digestion, prevents edema, alleviates sinus and bronchial congestion, and relieves arthritis symptoms. If you are taking any type of prescription drug while juicing, I would dissolve it in water or open the capsule if your doctor or health care professional approves.

If you have a major disease process, the massive amount of energy that is used for digestion can be directed toward healing. Over 95 percent of the nutritional value of raw juice is absorbed directly by the body. If your small intestine is inflamed, you absorb very few nutrients from your food. Look at your nails. If you do not observe "moons" above your cuticle, that means you are not absorbing nutrients and your current congestive diet may be starving your body of vital nutrients.

If you are a processed food addict, your body is acidic. Acids are very addictive, and people who eat an acid-rich diet with lots of meat have the largest challenge at first when switching to a raw juice regimen. A juice made of half a cabbage, one cucumber, and six celery stalks helps to neutralize those acids. My nephew quit smoking and started juicing. He has lost weight when most ex-smokers gain weight. He now finds more energy to exercise and enjoy life. He had been gaining weight and was threatened by the onset of diabetes. Having watched his father struggle with diabetes, he now feels he has control over his life and his health. The incidence of obesity and subsequent type 2 diabetes has tripled in the last forty years. As your pH becomes more alkaline, the organs of elimination in the body begin to function better, and you begin to eliminate health-threatening toxins. The bile in the gallbladder begins to thin, and it flows better, resolving issues with thick, viscous bile and the resulting creation of stones. It is important for bile to flow because it rids the body of unhealthy fats, congested hormones, and biohazardous toxins and bacteria. If the bile in the liver does not flow freely and becomes congested, hormones, bacteria, and toxins are recirculated and disease processes ensue.

I have had many personal experiences with fasting, both with water and raw vegetable juice. While my four-day water fast left me with a great deal of energy, my favorite type of fasting is juice-fasting. Once a year we do a seven-day raw juice fast, generally in March. And now we fast one weekend a month. This year, we tried an experiment. We drank the same juice (Dr. Mitchell's Detox Juice Recipe) every day, two to three times a day. We made enough juice to last for three days, so we only had to wash the juicer once instead of three times. At night, we had strained potassium tea with celery, broccoli, or garlic. We made enough potassium tea to last two nights, and refrigerated part of it. This made the fasting experience easier. We added one package twice daily between times of a powdered vitamin C drink that contained a full complement of other vitamins and minerals (Emergen-C Lite with MSM—the product is best in the "lite" form). This was added to ensure a balanced blood sugar level, since we were both working the same schedule as we always had. We found we had lots of time on our hands, and our grocery bill was about $50 a week for both of us juicing organic. I lost eleven pounds (5 kg) in seven days. We did decide that it would be better for most people to mix up the recipes and prepare two or three types of juice to keep from getting bored.

This chapter is primarily about raw juicing and the use of fiber-rich smoothies in general, but contains some tips on fasting and cleansing with juices as well. Please keep in mind that juicing is vital to restoring health. Not only are the enzymes important, but the vitamins, minerals, and trace elements found in raw fruits and vegetables are essential. Since our soils are so depleted, juicing allows us to get more of these vital nutrients into our body at one time without all the chewing. A bunch of romaine lettuce is reduced to half a cup (100 ml). Most people would not feel inspired enough to eat that much romaine at one sitting. A blender smoothie allows for extra fiber, which assists the colon in its cleansing process. But juicing provides more room for the vitamins and minerals alone, giving you access to the soul of the plant, so to speak.

It is also important to remember proper pH balance when preparing juices and smoothies. Greens are a major player in the creation of juice or a smoothie. You may mix and match the greens to suit your taste or detoxification or nutritional needs. So three-fourths of a good smoothie or juice recipe will contain greens (lettuces, kale, beet tops, collards, and even celery) of some kind. Nearly one-fourth of your recipe will contain fruit of some kind. For detoxification, I especially like beets, dandelion greens, ginger, or burdock root (also found in Asian markets as gobo) added to the juicing process. Pears are useful if you have a tendency for constipation. Apples help you achieve a good night's sleep, the pectin assisting in the absorption of serotonin. I am not particularly fond of citrus fruits in our juice or smoothie recipes, but they might have their place in yours if you need them. I also do not feel that "protein powders" are very useful at all. They are not raw. If you feel you need to use a protein powder, I would use one with a hempseed base. Excessive use of whey protein powders may leech calcium from the bones.

Vitamins are found in abundance in raw fruits and vegetables for juicing. Vitamin A–rich foods for juicing include carrots, spinach, cabbage, celery, and oranges. Adding a tablespoon of flaxseed oil to your juice ensures the absorption of vitamin A. Vitamin K and the B vitamins are found in abundance in spinach and the dark leafy greens: these include B_1, B_2, B_3, B_5 (found in cabbage), B_6, folic acid, biotin, and inositol (also found in cabbage). Vitamin C is found in those same greens as well as in citrus fruits.

The mineral content in raw juices makes them a good choice for detoxification and rebuilding, as noted below:

Calcium prevents inflammation and bolsters metabolism. It can be found in all dark greens, especially kale. It is also found in larger amounts in watercress, cabbage, and turnips. Carrots, lemons, and tangerines also contain lots of calcium.

Important for nerve and muscle function, and great to reverse restless leg syndrome, *potassium* is found in most leafy green vegetables, like spinach, parsley, dandelions, and kale. It is also abundant in potatoes, celery, grapes, tangerines, and lemons.

Sodium for cellular transport is found mostly in beets, kale, celery, dandelions, carrots, cherries, peaches, and tomatoes.

Magnesium is essential for the heart, muscles, and metabolism, and soothes nervous irritability. Magnesium is rich in raspberries, lemons, beets, endive, and apricots.

Phosphorus is important for bone formation as well as brain and nerve function. It exists in abundance in grapes, tangerines, raspberries, spinach, beet tops, carrots, cabbage, watercress, and kale.

Iron, which plays a key role in cellular oxygenation as part of hemoglobin, is found in spinach, apricots, parsley, wheatgrass, and beet tops.

While reviewing the above foods, which are high in minerals, we find the superstars of juicing: Kale is high in calcium, potassium, sodium, and phosphorus; beets (with beet tops) are high in calcium, potassium, sodium, magnesium, and phosphorus. Celery is high in sodium and potassium. Spinach is rich in iron, phosphorus, potassium, and calcium. Grapes are high in potassium and phosphorus. Carrots are high in calcium, sodium, and phosphorus.

Trace elements are also essential for health and immune function. Zinc is present in apples, pears, kale, carrots, lettuce, and asparagus. It is essential for the prostate, nerves, and immune functioning. Recent research has indicated that anorexia nervosa patients may benefit from consuming large amounts of zinc-rich foods or supplementing with zinc until they are able to taste a metallic taste when drinking liquid zinc tally. Iodine may be present in oranges and spinach, but only if iodine is in the soil for these to absorb that nutrient. Iodine helps the thyroid gland and supports metabolism. Copper, which is present in kale, potatoes, and asparagus, promotes the absorption of iron and benefits the brain and nerves. Manganese, found in apricots, oranges, spinach, romaine, kale, oranges, and strawberries, bolsters the reproductive processes.

On days when I am not teaching or in the clinic, we often add a large clove of raw garlic to our juice. I know of patients who add about a tablespoon (15 ml) of onion as well. Both garlic and onions contain the active constituent allicin, which some believe has antibiotic or immune-enhancing properties.

Garlic, a great bowel cleanser, also ameliorates gas and kills *Candida albicans*. Garlic is also known to reduce cholesterol and therefore promote vascular and heart function.

If you'd like, you might also use herbal teas as a base for blending smoothies. For example, if you have trouble with gas or flatulence, you might add calendula or fennel tea to your smoothie. See Chapter 20, on beverages, for added insights.

The superstars for juicing should be a part of every recipe daily. If you have a disease or disorder, you might consider the following nutrient-based additions to your juicing or smoothies:

Acid reflux: Juice raw cabbage. Drink 8 ounces (227 g) as often as needed. Reflux is often caused by too little hydrochloric acid in the stomach, rather than too much.

Anemia: A viable folk remedy is to cut up 1–2 beets and let them steep in 4 glasses of purified water overnight. Strain the water and drink throughout the day. Nettle tea is also useful as a bioavailable iron source.

Asthma: Juice a clove of garlic with carrots, small potatoes, beets, and a bit of greens. A teaspoon (5 ml) of lemon juice twice daily, followed by a swish of the mouth with warm water to protect the enamel is helpful.

Blood cleansing and thinning: Blood is always thinner after two weeks of juice cleansing. I feel that beets are a great blood cleanser. Dark juices from grapes, beets, and blueberries help to increase the circulation and production of red blood cells.

Cancer: Avoid carrots and citrus. Use celery, parsley or cilantro, spinach, ginger and 1/2 Granny Smith apple.

Constipation: Juice spinach, watercress, 1 clove of garlic, 1 tablespoon (15 ml) of onion, carrots, cucumber, beets, and celery. Try the "beet transit test." Eat one-half shredded raw beet and watch your eliminations to see how long it takes before your stool looks red. If it is more than 30 hours, your transverse colon is sluggish and may need some added stimulation. Eating more fiber in a smoothie is good, or drink flaxseed or Smooth Move tea.

Diabetes: Best produce to juice for diabetes is bitter melon, cucumbers (these help with insulin), raw green beans, parsley, celery, watercress, romaine, one clove of garlic, or a tablespoon (15 ml) of onion. I also suggest a tablespoon

(15 ml) of organic cinnamon added to your juice to bolster the power of insulin. While bitter melon tastes, well, bitter, combining it with carrot and apple will help.

Gallbladder, Liver: Juice grapes, carrots, and beets and a few springs of dandelion leaf. Artichoke leaf is also useful for ailments of the gallbladder, but it's bitter and therefore good for the gallbladder. Juice of pears is good for patients with gallstones.

High Cholesterol: Juice apple, romaine or watercress, grapefruit (if you're not taking a heart medication), blueberries (may be frozen if they're not in season) and one clove of garlic. Alfalfa tea is also useful.

High blood pressure: Potassium-rich vegetables help to remove accumulated salt from the tissues. A juice fast of three weeks could be very beneficial to a person with high blood pressure.

Joints: Joint function can be greatly improved by consuming carrots, beets, alfalfa sprouts, small potatoes (potassium-rich), grapes, and celery. If you decide on citrus fruits, eat them only occasionally.

Kidney: Lemons, juiced, help to dissolve uric acid stones. This bit of information is also helpful for people with gout. I suggest that you squeeze a half of lemon into an 8-ounce (227 g) glass of warm water and drink it first thing in morning. If you're brave, you might try juicing a small slice of horseradish with watercress, carrot, and celery. I would avoid the darker green leafy vegetables like kale and spinach because they contain oxalates that stress the kidneys. Teas: Corn silk, uva ursi, shave grass, gravel root, marshmallow root, or oatstraw.

Muscle twitches: Whether it is your eye that twitches or your legs at night, you could benefit from potassium. Juice turnips. A potassium broth tea made from organic potato skins generally helps. Scrub and soak in vinegar water 8 medium potatoes. Peel these, leaving the skin thick, and boil the skins in a quart (1 liter) of water for 10 minutes. Let them steep for another 10 minutes and strain. Drink a warm cup daily, especially at night during juice fasting. *Optional:* You may boil this brew with 6 cloves of garlic and or a cup (200 ml) of parsley.

Peptic ulcers: Juicing raw cabbage has been proven effective in healing peptic ulcers in less than a week.

Skin: Bernard Jensen, D.C., Ph.D., calls the skin the "third kidney." It is the largest organ of detoxification. For skin eruptions or rashes, juicing red grapes, beets, spinach, cucumber, and carrots seems to help. Keep in mind that most skin problems are rooted in a deeper toxic issue inside the body, unless it is an allergic reaction or contact dermatitis. Skin problems usually get worse before they get better. Consuming lots of water also helps.

Stomach problems: Juice carrots, tomatoes (although current research indicates that tomatoes as a nightshade are best cooked), celery, small potatoes, and cabbage. Cabbage juice is useful for stomach ulcers or *H. pylori*. I also like apple, lemon, and ginger to assist with digestion, if you have no problems with high blood pressure.

Thyroid: Our soils just do not contain iodine anymore. We add a sheet or two of nori to all our smoothies because it is tasteless. A tablespoon (15 ml) of soaked and strained kelp or dulse might be added to juice. Radishes contain a sulfur compound called raphanin that keeps the production of thyroid and the peptide hormone calcitonin in normal balance. With adequate amounts of raphanin circulating in blood plasma, the thyroid won't under- or overproduce these two hormones. This makes the tangy red radish a star when it comes to balancing the thyroid and treating thyroid diseases and Graves' disease. The sulfur amino acids in radish juice help break up fat deposits in the liver as well. Juice 1/2 cup (100 ml) sliced radishes with tops into carrot and apple juice.

Tonsils: Raw pineapple, carrots, watercress, a tablespoon (15 ml) of lemon, and beets are useful for cleansing the tonsils of infection. Especially when it comes to children, start with carrots, watercress or romaine, and raw pineapple and work into the other recommendations.

Weight: Juices containing celery, raw pineapple, dandelion leaf, grapes, parsley, lemon, and cucumber are very useful for bringing your weight down. If you do a juice fast for only one week, you can lose excess pounds, but juice-fasting for three weeks is even better. This helps to reset your system and give the colon a rest so that inflammation may heal.

A suggestion for additional benefit would be to add wheatgrass or cold herbal teas to your smoothies, instead of ice or other liquids. Remember to drink plenty of purified water.

When we prepare to juice, we always slice a separate snack of pineapple, carrot, and orange juice for later on.

GROWING AND JUICING WHEATGRASS

Growing your own wheatgrass is not rocket science, and it gives you a sense of confidence and peace of mind that what you are drinking is fresh and organic. Wheatgrass juicers range in price from forty dollars for the plastic manual counter attachment like the Healthy Juicer to the one hundred dollar stainless Handy Pantry HJ Hurricane. Electric "screw" type all-purpose juicers like Samson, Omega, Kuvings, and Greenpower run from two hundred thirty to five hundred dollars. Our Samson is still working great after ten years.

Wheatgrass packs a punch when consumed alone or added to raw smoothies or juice. I recommend that you only drink one half ounce to one ounce at a time for a week until you get used to how you feel. I have heard that wheatgrass is like a blood transfusion, and it has been used to ameliorate the effects of blood toxicity in chemotherapy. Some people report a sense of euphoria from the kick of the oxygen and enzymes, while others may experience a mild headache. A wedge of orange or an ounce of orange juice is often recommended following one or two ounces (called "shots") of wheatgrass. For more information, see Ann Wigmore's *Wheatgrass Book* that was published in 1985.

Growing Wheatgrass in Trays or Pots

1. Purchase in bulk organic hard red winter wheat berries online or from your natural foods store. If it doesn't say *organic,* it was probably treated with pesticides, insecticides, or fungicides.

2. Rinse $1^1/_2$ cups (300 ml) of the wheat berries, place them in a glass bowl, and cover with purified water (to $^1/_2$ inch [13mm] over the berries) for 12 hours or overnight. Put in a cool, dark place (not the refrigerator) and place a cover or lid over the top.

3. Strain and rinse the soaked wheat berries and scatter over organic soil that is $1^1/_2$ to 2 inches (3.8–5 cm) deep in a tray or pot. If the soil is deeper than 2 inches (5 cm), the energy of the plant goes into the roots rather than the

leaves. Commonly used are 10 X 20 inch (25.5 cm x 51 cm) flats, but any pot or even a cafeteria tray works. Spray the surface of the soil well with a mister and spread the soaked wheat berries densely in a single layer. (*Optional:* Cover with a thin layer of soil—as thin as you can make it.) Cover the tray with a layer of non-bleached paper towels, spray until damp, and put in a dark cool place.

4. As wheat berries germinate and sprout, check for bread mold and wipe it off if you find it. Mist if the soil feels dry. Cover and put the tray back in the cool, dark place. You should be seeing roots and sprouts within a few days. If there are no leaves or roots sprouting within five to seven days, the seed may be too old.

5. When the sprouts are nearly 1 inch (2.5 cm) tall, uncover and mist with a strained seaweed sluice to feed the plants iodine. Continue to keep the trays uncovered, in indirect sunlight or under a grow light or full spectrum light bulb until the blades of grass split. This happens when they are about 3–5 inches (7.5–12.5 cm) tall. They need to be misted or watered every day with only purified water (no seaweed sluice).

6. Harvest the wheatgrass with scissors or a knife by cutting just above the roots. If there is any mold present, cut above it. Cut only what you need at one time. If the grass gets tall and starts to lean over, cut and place what is left in a glass storage container and put it in the refrigerator. Grass that is too old or has yellow tips tastes bad. You may harvest a second cutting from the stubble if you water the grass that has already been cut once.

7. Compost the roots by breaking the soil into pieces. Do not reuse the soil, since it is depleted.

8. Drink the juice within 20 minutes of juicing if possible. It can also be used in the bathtub as a half-ounce (14 g) rectal implant (introducing the juice into the rectum/colon via the hydro-colon therapy, baby nasal bulb, or enema) or as a vaginal douche in water. Liquid chlorophyll can be purchased and used as well.

9. The expelled pulp can be used for skin poultices, as a facial, or to assist in healing sunburned skin, rashes, boils, bruises, or cuts.

Recipes Including Wheatgrass

BEE-GEE SWEETIE

Blend the following together and drink: 1–2 ounces (28–57 g) of wheatgrass, 1 cup (200 ml) of sliced, peeled, cold pineapple, 1 cup (200 ml) of fresh or frozen blueberries, 1 cup (200 ml) of chilled apple juice, 1 tablespoon (15 ml) raw honey, stevia, or agave nectar. (May be frozen into cream pops in an ice cube tray. Add sticks before frozen for handles.)

GREEN LEMONADE

Blend the following together and drink: 1–2 ounces (28–57 g) of wheatgrass and 1 cup (200 ml) of lemonade made with 1 cup (200 ml) of ice, 1–2 raw lemons, and 1–2 tablespoons (15–30 ml) agave nectar, stevia, or raw honey.

MICRO-GREENS

Follow steps 1–5 above using any type of leafy, green, organic garden seed instead of wheatgrass. Keep the young plants under the grow light as they continue to grow to about three inches (7.5 cm) tall and has the size of tender leaves that you want. Harvest only what you need, and continue to gently water or mist the micro-greens until they are cut. It is best to allow them to grow until you are ready to eat or juice them, but like the wheatgrass, if the plants start to fall over or look too pale, you can cut and refrigerate them.

THE MISSING LINK

When I review the diet of patients who have received allopathic cancer treatments, I am always very concerned that the foods they continue to eat feed cancer rather than starves it. It is critical that oncologists and patients study and implement intelligent nutritional standards to assist in the healing of cancer. Most research advocates that cancer patients avoid sugar and animal products, including meat and dairy.

I would like to share this personal letter from one of my patients. Please keep in mind that naturopaths educate each individual patient, not necessarily focusing on a particular disease. Our approach is based on each individual, not a "shotgun" or body-harming approach that scorches the terrain to kill the enemy, but one that supports the body, mind, spirit, and emotions of each person. Traditional naturopaths follow the original and true Hippocratic Oath: "First do no harm."

> *Working with Dr. Mitchell has changed my life. Her compassion and support made it all possible for me to get well. The doctor's diagnosis of cancer . . . was scary but she let me know that wellness could be achieved with whatever path I chose for treatment, as well as a change in my junk food diet. She educated me about how food intake impacts your health. No other doctor in my life ever talked to me about my diet. We also did several detoxification modalities which included colonics, which I also believe helped to save my life. Dr. Mitchell educated me each and every step of the way. My wellness and health have been and continue to be a journey. I am extremely hopeful that I will achieve 100 percent wellness. I have already beaten cancer. What a blessing you have been to me, Dr. Mitchell. I am forever grateful and thank you and God bless.*
>
> —MM, RN, PLAINFIELD, ILLINOIS

MEAT CONSUMPTION AND CANCER RISK

The World Health Organization determined that dietary factors account for at least 30 percent of all cancers in Western countries. When cancer researchers started to search for links between diet and cancer, one of the most significant findings was that people who avoided meat were much less likely to actually develop the disease. Large studies in England and Germany showed that vegetarians were about 40 percent less likely to develop cancer than meat eaters.

Harvard researchers recently conducted a prospective analysis of 90,655 premenopausal women, ages twenty-six to forty-six, enrolled in the Nurses' Health Study II. They determined that the intake of animal fat, especially from red meat and high-fat dairy products during premenopausal years, is associated with an increased risk of breast cancer. Increased risk was not associated with vegetable fats. A review of carcinogenic compounds showed that certain cancerous compounds are distributed to the mammary gland. As a consequence, tests indicate that frequent meat consumption may be a high risk factor for breast cancer.

SUGAR CONSUMPTION AND CANCER RISK

"If you have cancer, you should stop eating sugar immediately." This was the sage advice of Otto Warburg, Ph.D. More than seventy years ago, Dr. Warburg won the Nobel Prize in medicine when he discovered that cancer cells require glucose (sugar) for growth. All cells have a requirement for glucose, but cancer cells consume as much as four to five times more glucose than normal, healthy human cells. In fact, cancer cells are unable to multiply rapidly without it. It is astonishing to me that this simple research hasn't become the basis for instruction in any cancer protocol. If you eat sugar, fructose, and sweet fruits, or drink soda, you are feeding cancer.

ALKALINIZE YOUR DIET

An acidic environment is cancer's favorite home. A balanced alkaline diet helps to maintain the proper pH balance of the blood. If blood becomes more acidic, then the body will deposit excess acid in another area of the body. As more acids are consumed, storage areas will increase in acidity and some cells will die. The dead cells themselves will then turn into acids. If cells adapt to an acidic environment, they survive by mutating into malignant cells. These are rogue cells that continue to thrive from the consumption of acid-forming, refined, processed, and fatty foods. Constipation becomes a problem, and from that congestion of fecal matter, the blood begins to recirculate hazardous toxins and hormones that are held too long in the colon.

TAKE AN INVENTORY

Take a hard look at your diet. If you feel an emotional grieving process in the awareness that what you are eating may be unhealthy, put the adult who makes good decisions in charge of revitalizing your daily diet. It is not a situation that can be winked at or ignored, especially if you have a major disease, such as cancer. What you eat is your responsibility. After several days on an alkaline diet, most people find that the old sugars, fats, and processed foods are not appealing at all. It only takes a few days to begin a new, healthy way of life that can be pain-free and healthy. Your health is worth it.

SPROUTED BROWN RICE MILK

Soak 2 cups (400 ml) short-grain organic rice overnight, rinse and blend with 6 cups (1,200 ml) of purified water. Strain and store in the refrigerator. Take 2 cups (400 ml) daily in a blender smoothie or on raw fruit or sprouted grains. This stimulates the appetite; it's especially useful for treating bone cancer. The grain strained out can be used with 1 tablespoon (15 ml) miso as a poultice (topical application) for inflamed tissue.

BRUESS CANCER FAST

A man named Rudolf Breuss created an anticancer juicing formula that reportedly helped thousands of people who had cancer. This juice blend was intended as a fast that was used by over 24,000 patients, many of whom later wrote to him recounting their positive results. Over a period of forty-two days, his patients drank small amounts of this juice and the only other thing they consumed was a tea blend containing nettle, St. John's wort, marigold, artemisia (wormwood), and monarda (bee balm). His intent was to starve out the cancer cells and create a hostile environment for them. Breuss, who died at the age of ninety-three, reported that he achieved a 96 percent success rate for the thousands of patients he was able to treat over thirty years of his practice. His formula contained carrots, which I feel would be better avoided in the case of cancer. His juice contained: 1 beet, 1 celery stalk, 1 carrot, $1/_2$ of a potato, and 1 radish.

MODIFIED BRUESS CANCER FAST

Ingredients

1 beet plus tops

2 celery stalks

2 small organic potatoes

2 chard leaves

2 chard leaves or 1 cup (200 ml) fresh cleavers. (Cleavers are found growing close to the ground in yards and near wooded areas and are valuable blood and lymphatic cleansers.)

$1/_2$ bunch of cilantro

1 radish

1 clove of raw garlic

Directions: Wash and soak all produce in vinegar water. Juice all ingredients above. Enjoy.

CHAPTER 13

How to Help Children Eat More Greens

> *It's bizarre that the produce manager is more important to my children's health than the pediatrician.*
> —MERYL STREEP, FOOD TRENDS FOR 2011, USATODAY.COM.

I have assisted many parents in introducing vital green foods into a child's diet. One of the best ways that I know to introduce good, raw, nutritious foods to children is to preload vegetables after a busy day of school, sports, or playtime activities. In the May 2010 issue of the *American Journal of Clinical Nutrition*, Barbara J. Rolls and colleagues determined that if you feed preschoolers generous amounts of vegetables—in this case, raw carrots—as their first course, they will eat more of them. The National Institutes of Health funded this research as a means to discover how to increase vegetable nutrition in children and thereby prevent childhood obesity. You can prepare vegetables ahead of time, but finger-food vegetables should always be available for children to snack on. One mother told me that her ten-year-old son ate only microwave popcorn, Sprite, and potato chips and had no room for vegetables or fruit. He never ate them, claiming that they would make him vomit. Parents need to offer only good foods to their children; they alone invest in their child's state of health, parents are responsible for good nutrition. Vegetables and fruit must come first and frequent, and health-robbing dead foods should never be part of a child's diet. Creating a transitional meal flow that allows preloading of organic fruits and vegetables could go something like this:

Gala, Braeburn, Fuji, or Granny Smith apple slices

Cucumber, celery, broccoli, or red pepper strips.

Sautéed kale or spinach with garlic topped with sesame seeds and lemon juice.

Black bean, lentil, or brown rice soup in vegetable broth with vegetables.

Organic baby spinach or spring greens salad with sea salt, olive oil, and lemon juice.

The last course could be baked tempeh or veggie burger.

An hour or two later, a blueberry banana smoothie could take the place of ice cream.

Another great idea is to have a child grow a vegetable garden. You may not have a garden plot, but you can use a flowerpot to grow a package of lettuce seeds or soak a bowl of alfalfa seeds to sprout. Another good idea is to plan a field trip to a local farmers' market or visit the produce section of a grocery store to field-test small bits of produce. I would suggest that children be offered a sample of any vegetables or fruit that pique their curiosity. If children have eaten mostly acidic foods, they are likely to reject alkaline-based foods at first. Alkalinizing the diet for younger children may take a few days or even weeks to merge into, and the more resistance there is, the more important it is for parents to be persistent. Excessively acidic foods, constantly consumed, are not good for anyone, but they create catastrophic issues for children. Another method to consider is food preparation. I suggest that a food processor be used to chop larger amounts of greens and vegetables into smaller-looking servings. A cup (200 ml) of processed spinach looks like two tablespoons (30 ml) rather than half a plate.

If children do not learn to eat organic vegetables, they will not have adequate vitamins, minerals, and enzymes that will allow them to properly detoxify the biohazards of life in the twenty-first century. Without vitamins, minerals, and enzymes, children will become lethargic, anxious, and depressed. If they are not able to detoxify all the xenotoxins that threaten their biological well-being, they may eventually develop an autoimmune disorder or be at risk for a major disease. Dark greens are metal binders that assist in the binding and elimination of xenotoxins. This reduces the overall toxic burden. If a child's sensitive body is incapable of sustaining some semblance of a vibrant life, he may even eventually be incapable of reproduction. If you are a parent who is unknowingly neglecting to ensure that your children are eating vegetables daily, you are placing them sooner or later at risk of a major disease. If your children love sugar, breads, pasta, cheese, and meat, their bodies are probably bioacidic. An acid body leaves them emotionally, mentally, and physically at a disadvantage for the rest of their lives. No one teaches you the vital importance of eating green vegetables daily. I have been able to help parents reverse major mental and physical health challenges in their children simply by adding six child-appropriate servings of fresh vegetables as well as two servings of fruit daily to their diet. Bone density and calcium absorption are enhanced by dark greens. It is sad that parents feel they are depriving their children if they neglect to regularly serve them the deadly "whites." In her book *12 Steps to End Your Addiction to Cooked Foods,* Victoria Boutenko states, "Throughout history, whenever humans discovered an addictive substance, they never voluntarily stopped using it. Bread, milk, meat, sugar, and salt are probably the most addictive of all common foods. Research indicates that sweet receptors in the mouth are coupled to brain areas that release endogenous opiates—those natural morphine-like chemicals that induce a sense of pleasure and well-being. The taste of sweet in itself is enough to activate pleasure centers in the brain." If children (or adults) resist eating vegetables, it is because their poor little bodies are far too acidic and sugar-addicted. Persevere, and jump-start the greening process with sliced cucumbers (see the recipe for "Cucumber Pizza" below), celery (stuffed with almond butter and topped with raisins, if you'd like), fennel, and red leaf lettuce. Use agave nectar from cactus as a sweetener. Have your children shop with you in the organic produce department or the farmers' market to let you know which veggies intrigue them; even if it is parsley or carrot tops, buy it and try it. Introduce a new vegetable weekly, and introduce it ten times in the upcoming months. As their bodies become more alkaline, they will be more interested in dark greens and less interested in sugars, dairy, red meat, and processed foods. "Match stick"–prepared vegetables are user-friendly and easily consumed by children. (See "Sticks" recipe below.) Juicing can also be an adjunct to the introduction of greens in the diet. Children may find half a Granny Smith apple juiced with cucumber, celery, and romaine lettuce a nice treat. Let them help with the juicing. Remember to prewash your veggies in apple cider vinegar or veggie wash and store in ziplock bags with a sheet of damp paper towel.

I want to clarify what I mean by organic vegetables, enzymes, and toxic metal and chemical binders. In her latest book, *Green for Life,* Victoria Boutenko compares the vitamin and mineral content of organically grown vegetables to that of "conventional" vegetables. (I have a problem with the word *conventional;* it implies that this is what has always been. Prior to the chemical age following World War II, the "conventional method" of growing foods was pesticide-, herbicide-, GMO-, and toxic-free.) In many cases, conventional vegetables have little or no nutrient value because they are grown in depleted soils and forced through genetics to grow so quickly that the plant does not absorb vitamins and minerals from the sun and soil. Add to that the toxic ingestion of each plant's dose of chemical pesticides and herbicides. With cancer in this country occurring at a rate of nearly one in every two people, eating organic vegetables may help in preventing cancer by binding metals and xenotoxic chemicals already present in the body; eating organic foods also prevents the further addition of chemical residues that are an unwanted byproduct of conventional produce. Enzymes are present in raw fruits and vegetables. While they are affected during the digestive process by gastric acids, they are reassimilated in the small intestine, where they provide necessary energy and digestive absorption. Enzymes help the regenerative process of all muscles and nerves and reverse premature aging. If you are enzyme-depleted from consuming a too-dead diet, your body will "rob Peter to pay Paul." In order to perform its daily life tasks, your body will pull enzymes from the heart and the pancreas. Year after year, this depletion takes its toll on your tissue integrity. Heart disease and diabetes may follow. Remember that the adult in the family knows that health cannot be dictated by the least informed or most addicted member of the family. Try to include a rainbow of vegetables and fruits soon after you focus on the addition of greens, which are high in lutein and indoles (phytonutrients that boost the body's ability to rid itself of cancerous cells.) Avocados are brain- and heart-healthy, containing more vitamin E than any other fruit. Blue and purple foods contain anthocyanins and phenolics, which lower the risk of some cancers and have anti-aging benefits. The white of onions and garlic contain allicin, which was used to treat heart disease and as a natural antibiotic in previous centuries. Small potatoes contain lots of potassium, and mushrooms contain selenium. Yellow and orange produce contains vitamin C as well as carotenoids and bioflavonoids for heart, vision, and immune health. Red vegetables and fruit contain lycopene and anthocyanins that promote heart, memory, and urinary health, as well as helping to prevent cancer.

Part of the problem with acidic, dead, sugared, and processed foods is that they eventually cause inflammation in the colon. One problem that may develop from this inflammation is gluten-induced enteropathy, or gluten intolerance. There has been conclusive evidence linking gluten intolerance to both type 1 juvenile diabetes as well as multiple sclerosis. Edema or constipation may also be an issue. Yeast loves to grow in the cool dampness created by inflammation and sluggish eliminations, and parasites find a habitat where they can grow and reproduce without excessive disturbance. The disease process is setting in, and it is not long before the immune system is so over-taxed that an infection can develop somewhere in the body. Throw in some stress and antibiotics to destroy the invading bacteria and pathogens, and you now have a colon that is fully engaged in a catastrophic disease syndrome. The individual feels tired, irritable, bloated, unable to think straight or remember or retain anything, and knows that something somewhere inside is not very happy. It takes many months of enzyme-rich nutrition as well as rebuilding the friendly flora with probiotics before the body feels the trickle of health returning. Why not prevent this from happening to you or your loved ones? Start with good nutritional education provided by a source other than one with an economic prejudice. We are biological beings who need biological rather than chemically created, processed and frozen foods. Select the best the good green earth has to offer; organic foods definitely taste better. Vibrant health comes with every choice you make about what your children eat. Junk food takes away from health, organic vegetables and fruit add enzymes and energy to their life. I find that often adults who make poor food choices for themselves teach their children to do the same. It does not take a lot of work to cut an apple or rip open a bag of romaine lettuce and wash it, yet weekly I hear how hard produce is to prepare. Once upon a time, all vegetables were organic. Once upon a time, we lived in a country where people could expect their children to be healthy. If children do not love vegetables, it may be because their blood is too acidic; their yeast and parasites want to be fed; or they are addicted to sugar. Are you their health solution or the biggest part of the problem? Who buys the food? Make green, organic choices so your children can grow up healthy. Be persistent, patient, and make good decisions. Be an active voice in creating organic, nutritious, vegetable-based foods in school lunch programs, or send a cool pack with nutritious, delicious food choices prepared with your love at home.

ADD, ADHD, AND FAILURE TO THRIVE: SUGGESTIONS FOR PARENTS

Children can only focus mentally, thrive, and grow if their bodies are able to absorb vital nutrients. There are several reasons why absorption of nutrients is compromised and children fail to thrive and suffer their entire lives. To be a good parent is to offer your child nutritious food.

1. Children are offered processed, dead foods on a daily basis.

   - This robs the body of enzymes, and the body is forced to steal enzymes from the pancreas and heart just to digest food and for fundamental daily activities. Diabetes or hypoglycemia may result.

   - Processed foods, which are chemically designed to be highly addictive, replace nutrient-rich foods.

   - Because processed foods are full of sugar, corn, and wheat, and lack fiber found in vegetables, constipation and inflammation result.

2. They develop food intolerances from overeating difficult-to-digest, dead, fiber-free foods. Some children even shun foods because the resulting inflammation causes so much tissue damage that it hurts to eat. Food intolerances also cause failure to thrive or excessive weight issues.

   - Gluten is now processed with hexane and formaldehyde. It is a chemically created, nonbiological substance. Gluten has been linked to ADHD and type 1 juvenile diabetes. Chemically created flours are causing disease.
     ° Test gluten intolerance online $99. www.enterolab.com.
     ° Consider brown rice or quinoa pasta, UDI's bread, Pamela's gluten-free pancake and baking mix, breads from Anna muffin mixes, Namaste pizza crust, Mary Gone Crackers, or almond crackers. Gluten-free frozen products are available.

   - Dairy products from cows are difficult to digest. I suggest sheep or goat cheeses or milks made of almond or coconut; no soy products. See www.notmilk.com for more information about dairy. Encourage more water!

3. Children are not eating enough raw, green leafy vegetables. These are the calcium-rich body detoxifiers that are essential to a healthy life. You can get them via smoothies, in salads, or on GF sandwiches; process them in food processors; or add them to soups. If children do not like greens it is because they have not been offered them enough. Leafy greens are a must! An 8–10-year-old should have 2 cups (400 ml) of spinach or baby greens daily. Also a cup (200 ml) of vegetables like broccoli, cauliflower, kale, collards, celery, and cucumber, and another cup (200 ml) of green beans, peas, or edamame. The formula daily for all noninfant children is 6 of their fist-sized servings of vegetables ($^1/_2$ of which are raw); 2 servings of fruit, 1 of which is an apple; 1 serving of starchy foods like brown rice, sweet potatoes, or small potatoes; and 1 serving of protein-rich legumes like lentils or beans. Three times a week, a light meat like chicken or turkey or fish, and 1 time a week red meat (serving size a deck of cards or smaller). The key to a healthy alkaline lifestyle is 6-2-1-1 daily. It is also an outline for nutrients for a child's growth and development. Essential fatty acids found in avocado or added to the diet daily as flax oil mixed in salad dressings or smoothies are also helpful.

- Smoothie daily: 4 leaves of romaine or 1 cup spinach, 3 crunchy vegetables like 1 each of carrot, celery stalk, and 3 inches (7.5 cm) of cucumber. Add 1 cup of almond or coconut milk or water and 1 T of tahini or almond butter. May add agave nectar, $^1/_2$ banana, and a teaspoon of cinnamon.

- Pre-load vegetables or fruit after school or before meals.

4. Eliminate all soda pop or sweet drinks. Water for hydration: make sure they drink it! Soda leeches calcium from bones and causes blood sugar, weight, inflammation, liver, and malabsorption problems.

5. Avoid excessive animal protein. Elevates kidney stress, leeches calcium from the bones, and creates constipation problems as transit time is increased. It displaces nutrient-dense, easy-to-digest fruits and vegetables.

CHILD-FRIENDLY RECIPES

CUCUMBER PIZZA

Ingredients

1 medium-sized cucumber

Optional toppings: Chopped black or green olives, chopped fresh basil, thinly sliced or chopped tomatoes, chopped red pepper, dill, Italian spices, garlic salt

Directions

Cut the cucumber in half and chop gently at the top of the cuts on each side. Rub these two cuts together vigorously until they foam. (This removes the bitterness from the inside of the cucumber.) Rinse off the foam. Slice the cucumber into rounds. On top of the rounds place any or all of the optional toppings. Put on a plate and munch!

NO MORE RANCH DIP

Many people like to dip vegetables in white dairy dressing. Make your own healthful nondairy dip instead.

Ingredients

¼ cup (50 ml) raw almond butter

6 tablespoons (90 ml) olive or roasted sesame oil

1 tablespoon (15 ml) lemon juice

1 tablespoon (15 ml) agave nectar

Herbs to season

Directions

Stir all ingredients together.

STICKS

Ingredients

Red peppers, snow peas, cucumbers, carrots, squash,
celery, jicama (pronounced he-KA-ma [most kids love this]),
sweet potatoes, and any vegetable (or fruit)
that can be sliced into matchsticks.

Directions

Julienne any of the above vegetables. If desired, add a dressing (below) or leave the sticks plain as snacks. Don't be afraid to mix in some ants (raisins), walnuts, or raw cacao.

DRESSING

Ingredients

1 cup (200 ml) extra-virgin olive oil (fresh)

2–4 tablespoons (30–60 ml) toasted sesame oil

4 tablespoons (60 ml) Bragg Aminos

4 tablespoons (60 ml) either agave nectar, raw honey, or almond butter

4 tablespoons (60 ml) lime or lemon juice

Italian herbs added to your taste

Directions

Stir all ingredients together.

Variations: Add garlic (optional). You may also use lemon instead of lime, but it gives the dressing a different taste.

OREOOOS

A great snack for after school.

Ingredients

Raw sweet potatoes, yams, or apples

Almond butter

Directions

Peel and thinly slice whichever ingredients you choose. Butter the slices with almond butter, and top with another slice. Consider mixing the apples with the sweet potatoes.

RAW MASHED POTATOES
(ADAPTED FROM NOMI SHANNON, THE RAW GOURMET)

Ingredients

$1/2$ head cauliflower

1 tablespoon (15 ml) lemon juice

$1/4$ cup (50 ml) extra-virgin olive oil

1 small clove garlic or $1/2$ teaspoon (5 ml) garlic salt

$1/2$ teaspoon (3 ml) poultry seasoning

$1/2$ teaspoon (3 ml) Bragg Aminos or a dash of sea salt

If you have it, add $3/4$ teaspoon (4 ml) psyllium powder

Directions

Wash in veggie wash and rinse all ingredients. Place them in a food processor with an S-blade or in a blender. Blend until smooth. Serve.

ALIVE IN 5

Raw Gourmet Meals in Five Minutes, by Angela Elliott, has many awesome easy snack and vegetable ideas that are quick to create. Have fun. And remember my personal favorite below!

FRUIT ICE DREAM

Ingredients

1 bag frozen organic fruit (blueberry is my favorite)

$1/2$ cup (100 ml) ice, almond, or oat milk (or water with 1 T of almond butter)

1 frozen chopped banana (We freeze any bananas that are getting too ripe
and use them in a smoothie.)

Directions

Blend until smooth and creamy. (I add 2 tablespoons [30 ml] flax oil)

Another variation of Fruit Ice Dream follows.

P.B. & J. SMOOTHIE

Ingredients

½ cup (100 ml) almond or coconut milk

4 tablespoons (60 ml) almond butter

4 tablespoons (60 ml) cacao nibs

1 cup (200 ml) frozen raspberries or strawberries

1 frozen banana

Directions

Blend all ingredients until smooth.

Variations: You may also add cinnamon or vanilla. I also add to this 2
tablespoons (30 ml) flax oil.

ORANGE MONKEY SMOOTHIE

Ingredients

1 cup (200 ml) frozen orange juice

1 frozen banana (slice and freeze bananas when they start to turn)

¼ cup (50 ml) hemp, sesame, almond, or coconut milk

½ cup (100 ml) frozen organic berries of your choice: mixed, blueberries, strawberries, or
raspberries

Directions

Blend all ingredients.

JAME'S APPLE AND WORM JUICE

Ingredients

1 cucumber

1 apple

$\frac{1}{2}$ cup of purified water

Directions

Remove seeds from apple, chop it with cucumber. Put in blender with water. Blend until smooth.

BANANA MANGO PUDDING

Ingredients

1 cup (200 ml) soaked cashews or macadamia nuts

1 fresh banana or $\frac{1}{2}$ cup frozen banana chunks

1 mango, peeled and sliced, or $\frac{1}{2}$ cup (100 ml) frozen mango chunks

2 tablespoons (30 ml) agave nectar or raw honey

1 teaspoon (5 ml) gluten free vanilla

$\frac{1}{2}$ cup of water

Directions

Blend all ingredients with water until smooth. Chill and keep in the refrigerator.

Variation: Add 2 tablespoons (30 ml) coconut milk. You may also top this dish with blueberries.

I often suggest to parents that children might have to taste a new vegetable at least ten times before they find it appetizing. I also encourage them to use a food processor to chop raw greens fine so they are easier to eat and more seems like less. Six leaves of romaine or collards might easily macerate into half a cup (100 ml) of processed greens. Juicing is also fun for children if adults have the right attitude about it, and it can be a way to encourage the consumption of raw vegetable greens and fruits. Keep in mind that a twin-gear or centrifugal juicer allows you to keep and refrigerate the juice for up to three days without excessive loss of valuable enzymes so you have less time invested in cleanup weekly if you only juice twice a week, rather than every day. A six-year-old patient who suffered with Tourette Syndrome and hated vegetables was symptom-free after two weeks of drinking my raw juice recipe. This is not the first time I have been able to assist in healing the symptoms of Tourette's simply by altering the diet and adding in nutrient and enzyme-rich fruits and vegetables.

I would recommend six ounces (170 g) of one of my alkaline juices daily for children four to eight years of age; for nine- to twelve-year-olds, eight ounces (227 g). For teens and adults I feel that ten ounces (284 g) a day is most beneficial. The ginger in juice recipes helps warm the digestion of the cool, alkaline juice. In the winter and in colder climates, warming teas and ginger- and curcumin-rich chilies are good remedies for preventing what we call "cool dampness," which can escalate into a yeast problem. Warmth in the gut translates to better digestion and assimilation and enhanced immune function.

In another vegetable-resistant case, the mother of Laura, a very sick six-year-old diagnosed with ADHD, told me that her fussy daughter refused to eat vegetables and fruits. She would only eat boxed macaroni and cheese and chicken nuggets. These denatured, processed foods were robbing Laura of vital health. When living foods became her primary diet, Laura's health and behavior changed dramatically. It wasn't easy, but Laura's mom made the dietary change with her.

Teaching our children healthy eating habits is an important parental responsibility. Feeding children only what they want leads to disastrous consequences. Many so-called genetic diseases and disorders are more accurately the result of poor family eating patterns or food intolerances that run in families. Accurate nutritional information or intolerance testing could solve that nagging problem misdiagnosed as "genetic." Many laboratories will test you for dairy or gluten intolerance. Please be aware that an intolerance or sensitivity is not the same as a food allergy. One such laboratory that I refer patients to is Entero Lab (www.enterolab.com). By sending in a stool sample, a patient can soon have a report of food sensitivities. There are a growing number of people who are unable to tolerate gluten and or how it is chemically processed.

In my practice, it makes me very sad to see young children suffer with allergies, autoimmune disorders, or behavioral challenges because I know that most of these issues are diet-related and can be reversed or prevented. In my initial interview I often discover that these sick children refuse to eat vegetables or are never offered them. Their diets generally contain a blizzard of white biohazards: sugar, processed foods with white refined flours like pasta, and lots of ice cream, cheese, and dairy. In my early years of practice, I used to encourage what is called an elimination diet. I would tell parents that what their children are experiencing on the inside is manifesting on the outside in terms of actions, activities, or aggravated cellular response. I tell parents that they need to understand that they are purchasing acidic, toxic foods that should never be fed to anyone or anything in the family. I educate them about 4-3-2-1 eating: 4 raw, individual, fist-sized servings of leafy green vegetables, 3 varied other vegetables and starches, 2 fruits, and one nut or grain serving daily for pH-balanced nutrition. Adults always ask, "What are we going to eat?!" This is then followed by a litany of the usual industry-standard commercial information: "Doesn't milk do a body good?" "You can't buy anything without sugar or flour." But my personal favorite is "I'll never get my children to eat anything green." I offer to send in a hair sample to the lab for analysis of toxic elements, knowing that it will reveal a body that is overwhelmed by such toxic elements as mercury, antimony, barium, uranium, nickel, lead, and aluminum. I do this so that the parents can see on a laboratory printout what a lack of greens allows to remain or exist in the body. Without enzymes and green plant foods, the body is unable to bind and remove metals from the body. These toxins are biohazards that settle in the brain, the long muscles, the organs, the bones, and other places we would never want them.

SPECIFIC NUTRITIONAL NEEDS
FROM BIRTH THROUGH CHILDHOOD

Nutrition for Infants

About 35 percent of the four million babies born each year have a reflux difficulty in the first few months of their lives, and some might outgrow the condition before they are a year old. Some will not, however, and occasionally babies do not spit up but still have other symptoms. If the acid reflux is coming up and then going back down the esophagus, it could cause twice the problems as far as both pain and damage are concerned. I believe that when babies are fed processed cow or soy formulas, or formulas that have no enzymes, these formulas create reflux in children. A daily probiotic like Natren's Healthy Start or Pure Encapsulations Purebaby probiotic is always useful. If an infant is not breast fed, I would consider goat's milk, a liquid multivitamin, and plant-based DHA. Some parents include a bit of coconut oil internally as well as topically.

Six months is probably the earliest time to begin feeding that little infant any solid foods. Waiting until six months of age gives babies time to develop their digestive tract and immune system. This reduces the likelihood of allergies. Initial foods should be simple, natural, and puréed to promote digestion. The true flavors of food are best; avoid sweetened or salted foods, especially foods with refined sugar and refined flour. Avoid gluten. First foods may be puréed fruits and vegetables, one at a time, such as avocado or a small amount of mashed banana. Raw carrots contain beta-carotene, which is the safest form of vitamin A. Vitamin A is very good for babies because it helps improve the health of the eyes, the brain, and the skin. In addition, vitamin A also boosts the immune system and enhances the potency of other antioxidants like vitamins C and E. Vitamin E is found in many vegetables, such as green beans and carrots. This vitamin is good for eye and hair health. When introducing your baby to raw foods, be sure to start with one puréed food at a time and only feed your baby that particular food for one week. See how the baby responds to the new changes in her diet. If you see any signs that the baby is not ready for solid food, like a diaper or skin rash, switch foods immediately and try another type of vegetable for a week. Introducing raw foods into your baby's diet is an experiment in the beginning. The baby's system is new. Always introduce vegetables before fruit because fruit is more acidic, and you want your baby to develop a taste for greens first. Raw foods contain generous portions of enzymes and fiber. Both of these nutrients are critical for healthy digestion. Enzymes help your baby's body break down fats, proteins, and carbohydrates. Enzymes also bolster the entire metabolic process so that your baby gets the most from her food. Fiber is very beneficial because fiber regulates digestion. Fiber helps babies have much easier bowel movements and fewer stomach problems, like bloating. Fiber also bonds to everyday toxins that the baby is exposed to in the environment. Fiber absorbs these wastes and flushes them out of the body quickly. These foods, along with mother's milk, will provide the proper nourishment for this time of rapid growth.

Nutrition for Your Growing Child

From eight months to one year, babies may be more independent, adventurous, and enthusiastic about what they eat. They are willing to try more new foods. Breast milk consumption may be reduced, but it is still a regular source of nourishment. Infants may be weaned at this time, though many mothers will continue nursing for another year or more.

After one year, the infant's diet may change. The need for food to foster growth is less pressing now, as the rate of growth slows down. Offer only nourishing foods and avoid sweet treats—no sugar. At this age, children do well with green smoothies. These are any greens blended with some fruit and hemp seeds and flax oil. You can add soaked seaweed, spirulina, chlorella, sunflower lecithin, or coconut oil. Make sure you focus on leafy greens, so the child develops strong teeth and bones, and also enough fat and omega fatty acids for brain development.

Vitamin and Mineral Supplements for Children

When a vitamin formula is used, it is often a liquid supplement in the first years. For toddlers, the multiple should contain all the B vitamins, plus vitamins C, E, and A. Basic minerals, such as calcium and iron, as well as zinc, magnesium, manganese, and even a little chromium and selenium, may also be included. I suggest only natural, chemical-free supplements. Table 13-1 shows the levels of vitamins and minerals suggested for children from birth to two years old.

TABLE 13-1	DAILY REQUIRED NUTRIENTS—INFANTS AND TODDLERS		
	BIRTH–6 MONTHS	6 MONTHS–1 YEAR	1–2 YEARS
Calories	115 kilograms (kg)	105–110/kg	1,200–1,400 kg
Protein (grams)	2.2 grams (g)	2.0 g	22–25 g
Vitamin A	2,000 international units (IUs)	2,000 IUs	2,500 IUs
Vitamin D	400 IUs	400 IUs	400 IUs
Vitamin E	5 IUs	6 IUs	8 IUs
Vitamin K	15 micrograms (mcg)	25 mcg	30 mcg
Thiamine (B_1)	0.4 milligram (mg)	0.6 mg	0.8 mg
Riboflavin (B_2)	0.5 mg	0.7 mg	0.9 mg
Niacin (B_3)	6 mg	8 mg	10 mg
Pantothenic acid (B_5)	3 mg	3 mg	4 mg
Pyridoxine (B_6)	0.4 mg	0.6 mg	1.0 mg
Cobalamin (B_{12})	1.0 mcg	2.0 mcg	2.5 mcg
Folic acid	40 mcg	60 mcg	100 mcg

Biotin	50 mcg	50 mcg	50 mcg
Vitamin C	40 mg	60 mg	100 mg
Calcium	400 mg	600 mg	800 mg
Chloride	0.6 g	1.0 g	1.2 g
Chromium	50 mcg	60 mcg	80 mcg
Copper	0.7 mg	1.0 mg	1.5 mg
Fluoride	0.3 mg	0.6 mg	1.0 mg
Iodine	50 mcg	60 mcg	80 mcg
Iron	10 mg	15 mg	15 mg
Magnesium	70 mg	90 mg	150 mg
Manganese	0.7 mg	1.0 mg	1.5 mg
Molybdenum	60 mcg	80 mcg	100 mcg
Phosphorus	300 mg	500 mg	800 mg
Potassium	0.7 mg	1.0 mg	1.5 mg
Selenium	40 mcg	60 mcg	80 mcg
Sodium	0.3 g	0.6 g	0.9 g
Zinc	4 mg	6 mg	10 mg

GIVING CHILDREN THE NUTRITION THEY NEED

By eating real, live, whole foods, including lots of leafy greens, fresh vegetables, and fruit, as well as sprouted whole grains and legumes, children can get their necessary vitamins in the way that biological beings were meant to. This is the healthiest way. Vitamins occur in real foods in digestible forms that are the easiest for the body to absorb. One of the most important challenges of parenting is to provide healthy foods for children while helping to make eating these whole foods a pleasant experience.

Unfortunately, vitamin deficiency diseases are common among American children. Most children eating a standard American or junk food diet get suboptimal vitamins—levels low enough to adversely affect their health, their intellect, and their behavior. Because children are eating too many processed foods, they are getting suboptimal levels of at least thirteen nutrients. The poor standard diet of nonorganic fruits and vegetables provides minimal vitamins and nutrients, but contains health hazards of pesticides and herbicides. I am shocked that some children are failing to thrive. Their bodies are not responding to foodless foods. If children are not eating organic foods, their bodies may suffer malnutrition. For that reason, I encourage a liquid multivitamin with extra vitamin D as a supplement to the vitamins they get in their food.

While researching current information for a nutrition class that I was teaching, I read that Americans spend ninety cents of every food dollar on processed foods. Not only is this a waste of good money, but eating too much processed, bioacidic food is the first step toward most disease processes. There are grassroots campaigns in Canada to abolish many of the commercial products and processed foods that increase the probability of disease and ill health. Several types of produce grown in the United States are currently banned in Canada because they are considered a health hazard as a result of the chemicals they contain.

If we believe what we are told, we live in the best of all times because our technology and medical advances have afforded us limitless advantages and time to pursue the American dream. We are supposed to have more time for leisure since GE promised us that technology would replace our presence in the daily grind. In the 1950s, families purchased the can opener, boxed cake mixes, and technofoods to ensure a happy future, but in the process, we lost track of our recipes calling for whole foods, our kitchens, our gardens, our family tables, and the ability to experience the joy of sharing communication and co-creation as a community.

A technology-based diet contains food that plops out of a box or a can and is not nourishment, but most often generates internal pollution and toxic waste for the body to deal with. Food that does not nurture the body does one or two things to it: it robs the body of vitality as the body struggles to digest it and, if it is indigestible, these toxins lodge in the liver or in tissue as xenotoxins or internal pollutants. These foods include cholesterol-building trans fats, such as those in margarine and processed cheeses, and overprocessed, enhanced dead foods, such as those made with white flour and sugar. These substances create challenges for the organs and the lymphatic system, the blood, and the mental processes. An unbalanced or polluted liver may cause anger, fear, and depression. In short, we are trading our ability to make conscious and selective food choices to fatten a technology-based food industry just because we are not empowering ourselves to make a small change in our habits. Many of our bad food habits are influenced by commercial advertising. As we or our children sit and watch television in our spare time, with our health-stealing packaged foods, we feel more and more depressed. We gain a lot of weight. It seems like a syndrome of powerlessness, culminating, perhaps, in a disease like diabetes. We appear addicted to our lethargy, the easy or thoughtless way of dealing with food. We often open it and eat it, or drive through and throw it in our unprepared stomachs.

If you read the labels on food and soda pop, you find that you are unable to pronounce certain words that indicate laboratory modification of what once was whole food. Many people are not aware that current research links chronic diseases, such as fibromyalgia and chronic fatigue syndrome as well as diabetes, to technologically created sweeteners or high-fructose corn syrup. If you or your children drink "regular" soda, there are approximately seventeen teaspoons (85 ml) of sugar in one can of soda. I have seen children's ability to focus and remain calm increase in just one week by eliminating from their diet technology-based foods—soda pop, and sugar, in particular. Some of these same children were consuming at least a cup (200 ml) of sugar a day! No wonder they were bouncing off the walls in a constant brain fog, unable to think or sleep at night. Opportunistic *Candida albicans* yeast waits for sugar, and this yeast, like an internal dragon, demands to be fed. Aberrant behavior soon follows bad nutrition.

EMPOWERING OURSELVES TO MAKE SMART DECISIONS ABOUT FOOD

So the question remains: if we could turn back the clock to pre–World War II days, would we want to do so? We must empower ourselves to choose food wisely at all times. To fail to do so is not good body stewardship. We can make good food choices based on our own discernment and research. We must educate ourselves about good nutrition and change our lazy food habits. Washing organic vegetables for a meal does not require a great deal of time when compared to the time we spend as a nation watching television or driving miles for fast food. If we do not eat fresh, dark greens, such as broccoli, spinach, romaine, collard greens, kale, and dandelions, we miss out on one of the greatest nutritional benefits—the B vitamins. B vitamins have a great deal to do with mood, mental processes, endocrine hormones, and disease prevention. Avocado is also rich in B vitamins, beneficial oils, and essential fatty acids.

Vitamin C and beta-carotene are present in such wonder foods as carrots, raw oranges (not pre-bottled orange juice), and kiwi. Kiwi has more vitamin C than oranges. Vitamin C bolsters stress-reducing hormones.

Dairy as a food has many hidden concerns, including antibiotics, pesticides, and rBGH hormones that can cause lactation in women and precocious puberty in very young children. The government has increased the allowable blood and erythrocytes (pus) in milk products as well. See www.notmilk.com for further information. If you want to get calcium from a great source, look at what a cow does. She eats her greens. Broccoli is very rich in calcium and magnesium. The body truly does not require that much calcium. We are led to believe that osteoporosis comes from a lack of calcium in the diet, but the problem is actually one of absorption. The body needs vitamin K and biotin, intrinsic factors in the small intestine that allow the uptake of calcium into the bones. Dark green vegetables are rich in vitamin K, but because many Americans are not eating enough dark, leafy greens, calcium cannot be absorbed and is often shuffled off to the joints to cause lactic acid/calcium joint hypercalcification. Osteoporosis is also a byproduct of a sedentary lifestyle and comes from drinking too much soda pop or caffeine or eating excessive animal protein that leeches calcium from the bones. By walking just ten minutes a day, you will strengthen your bones.

Whenever I interview new patients, I get an immediate sense of food intolerance problems. Black bags under the eyes reflect dairy intolerance or "dairy shiners." One new patient was surprised when I inquired about her family history of diabetes, arthritis, constipation, and even colon cancer. How did I know? I knew just by looking at her. She claimed that she had had dark bags under her eyes since she was a child. I said that as a child she probably suffered from ear infections, acne, and perhaps respiratory infections too. All these are indications of a dairy intolerance. After just one month on a dairy-free diet, the dark bags disappeared and she had more energy than she ever believed possible.

Naturopathic medicine is all about wellness and the prevention of disease. The healthiest countries in the world value the efforts of doctors and health practitioners who keep their people free of a dependence on drugs. Insurance companies pay more for wellness appointments than for the treatment of disease. They have found that they save a great deal of money when they do so. If you do not have a true wellness doctor to help you achieve and maintain good health in today's world, I encourage you to find one.

CHAPTER 14

Raw Foods to Consider for the Healing of Disease

"The doctor of the future will give no medicine, but will interest his patients in the care of the human frame, in diet, and in the cause and prevention of disease."

—THOMAS EDISON, QUOTE TO FRIEND

According to the Law of Similars, we eat foods that treat the body part resembling that particular plant, fruit, or vegetable. Some examples of this are beets for blood, avocado for belly fat, and walnuts for the brain. These examples are just a beginning, offered for clarification only. The following list of conditions specifies foods or nutrients that are often deficient among those suffering from those condition and foods or nutrients that might help remedy the condition:

Addictions: To alcohol, cigarettes, and drugs. These three addictions cause depression and loss of years in the life span—a loss of up to ten to twelve years. Nutritional deficiencies common to those who are addicted include zinc; vitamins A, B, and C; plus selenium, magnesium, antioxidants, amino acids like L-carnitine and L-glutamine, probiotics, and essential fatty acids. Mushrooms are high in zinc, and I have found raw juice-fasting with lots of dark greens beneficial in detoxifying nicotine and overcoming the addiction of these substances.

Acid reflux, also known as gastroesophageal reflux disease (GERD): Drink 8 ounces (227 g) of freshly juiced cabbage as often as needed. Adjust the ileocecal and pyloric valves. The ileocecal valve is the junction of the small intestine and the ascending colon. It is found halfway on the diagonal between the naval and the right hip. I teach patients to massage deeply, three times counterclockwise, on the area that is tender in that location. It often feels like a tender knot. Then push toward the left hip. Repeat two more times until there is a gurgle or it is less tender. To find the pyloric valve, go directly under the base of the sternum and move to the left about one of your hand lengths. You should be under your left lowest rib. Palpate until you feel a tender spot, again like a knot. Massage deeply three times and push down. Pump the tender spot five times. Repeat the massage and pushing down two more times or until you feel a change in the tenderness or you hear a gurgle. Check these two valves once or twice a day or as needed. Resetting the ileocecal valve often assists with sinus trouble. Take enzymes or hydrochloric acid ten minutes before meals. Avoid gluten and nightshades like eggplant, tomatoes, and green peppers, or other possible reactive antigens in the diet.

Alzheimer's disease: Nutritional deficiencies and xenotoxins are common with Alzheimer's. Antioxidants, vitamins B_1 and B_{12}, zinc, amino acids, DHEA (a hormone that declines with aging), and melatonin are often deficient. Chlorella is very beneficial. I use a chelation method with EDTA and CoQ_{10} that assists in detoxifying metals such as aluminum. Avoid foods, cans, pans, and deodorants that contain aluminum.

Anemia: Parsley and grapes. Nettle tea or juice nettles. Black strap molasses.

Anorexia nervosa: Zinc deficiency is the latest concern. Four ounces (113 g) of liquid zinc daily until you discern the metallic taste. Eat zinc-rich raw foods daily or a nutritious raw foods diet, complete with all you can eat without worrying about gaining weight.

Asthma or *hypoxia:* Eat garlic, and avoid dairy. Do a homeopathic or herbal parasite detox for eighteen days, and eat one tablespoon of pumpkin seeds during that detox.

Belly fat: Eat avocado daily, together with a raw diet. Detoxify stress from your life as elevated cortisol has been linked to holding weight around the belly.

Benign prostatic hyperplasia: Saw palmetto tea or tincture daily as well as *Pygeum africanum* to relieve the symptoms of BPH. Raw diet.

Blood cleansing: Beets and tops, freshly juiced burdock, or cleavers, that prolific plant growing close to the ground in your backyard or by a wooded area.

Cancer: Sprouted brown rice milk. Bruess juice fast. Colon cleanse. Detoxification with alternative teas or tinctures. Parasite detox. See Hulda Clark's *The Cure for All Cancers.*

Chronic candidiasis: Garlic, fresh oregano, or Pau D'Arco tea. Gluten- and sugar-free or raw diet. Avoid fermented foods. Probiotics.

Chronic fatigue, fibromyalgia: A raw diet. No sweets. Avoid carrots. Yeast detoxification.

Constipation: Celery, spinach, and grapefruit juiced. Four prunes soaked in water and blended or eaten 2–3 times a day until you see results. Drink 6 ounces (170 g) every 2 hours. Or try Epsom salts in water: 1 tablespoon (15 ml) to 8 ounces (227 g) of water. Drink every 2 hours until you see results.

Cystitis: Juiced celery and pomegranate juice, or juiced cranberries. Agrimony, marshmallow, Uva ursi, nettle tea blend.

Diabetes mellitus: A raw diet. See the DVD by Gabriel Cousens, titled *Reversing Diabetes in Twenty-One Days.* Twenty-five percent of Americans over the age of 60 have type 2 diabetes, a condition some believe is reversible by switching to a raw diet. It is now an epidemic related to enzyme-depleted, sugar- and fat-laden processed foods.

Diarrhea: Carrots and blackberries juiced or blended. One-half banana. Black walnut hull tincture: place 4 milliliters (a dropper's full) in water every 4 hours and drink. Arsenicum alb., 30X or 30 C potency. Arsenicum is a homeopathic remedy. Take 10 pellets every 15 minutes until the symptoms improve. Then take every 2–4 hours.

Endometriosis: Iodine-rich sea vegetables and a raw diet.

Eczema: See *Psoriasis* or *eczema.*

Fibrocystic breasts: Iodine-rich sea vegetables. Lugol's Iodine applied topically to breast cyst at night before bed. Do not wear an underwire bra—ever.

Gallstones: Celery juice, black cherry juice or smoothies. Flaxseed tea. Do a gallbladder flush.

Gout: A raw diet, no animal or acidic foods. Juice turnips or raw juice fast for seven days.

Hair loss (allopecia): Inflammation in the colon may be a problem. Taking L-glutamine or biotin is helpful as it is created in the small intestine as an intrinsic factor. Sea vegetables.

Hiatal hernia: A hiatal hernia is an anatomical abnormality, present in approximately 50 percent of the population, caused by inflammation or gastric reflux. Part of the stomach is forced to protrude through the diaphragm and up into the chest. I have had patients report having heart attack symptoms that were actually hiatal hernia reactions to acid reflux or foods like raw tomatoes. I really like 1 tablespoon (15 ml) of slippery elm in 10 tablespoons (1,200 ml) warm water for assistance with hiatal hernia and/or 3 ounces (85 g) of aloe vera juice twice a day. Avoid nightshades like tomatoes, green peppers, and eggplant.

High blood pressure: Carrot, celery, and parsley juice. Take 200 mg of CoQ_{10} as ubiquinol daily.

High cholesterol: Insulin tells the liver to increase production of cholesterol. The liver produces 82 percent of blood cholesterol. Carbohydrates increase our cholesterol level. Eating more raw greens increases the alkaline nature of the blood. Citrus fruits and apples are high in pectin that helps to lower cholesterol.

h Pylori bacteria in the stomach: Haritaki or triphala, berberines like Oregon grape. All are dried fruit or herbs.

Hypothyroid symptoms: Nutrient-rich sea vegetables and chlorella are essen iodine. Also, fluoridated water, metals in the system, parasites, gluten, and pesticides may be stressors of the thyroid. Pure water and a good detox for parasites or metals might be useful.

Hypoglycemia: Carry almonds mixed with raisins with you to snack on frequently. Eat at least five meals a day, and start your morning with a smoothie with almonds and avocado.

Irritable bowel syndrome: Raw coconut milk, a raw diet, or lightly steamed vegetables to transition to a raw diet.

Insomnia: Lettuce and celery juice daily. More magnesium, B_6, and an apple daily. I have found L-tryptophan (600 mgs. 1-3 capsules) very helpful and hour before bedtime. If that does not help, 5HTP (100 mg. 2 caps) is beneficial.

Kidney stones: Herbal tea mixture of gravel root, marshmallow, and hydrangea—2 tablespoons (30 ml) to a quart (1 liter) of hot water. Steep overnight and strain. Store excess in refrigerator. Drink slowly, 1 cup (200 ml) daily. Avoid black tea and darkest greens, like spinach, which contain oxalates.

Menopause (for symptoms of menopause, which is not a disease): No soda or red meat. A raw diet. Lachesis mutus homeopathic remedy: 10 pellets as needed for hot flashes, or 10 pellets 4–6 times daily to prevent the onset of hot flashes. Exercise and magnesium-rich foods.

Migraines: Sea vegetables, magnesium, trace minerals, a gluten-free raw diet. Raw fennel, especially juiced.

Multiple sclerosis: Vitamins: 500 mg B_6, and 500 mg flush-free niacin, B_{12} 5,000, 100,000 IU beta carotene, CoQ_{10} 200 mg daily, 100 mg 7KetoDHEA (androgens do not translate into estrogen or testosterone), 5,000 mg ascorbate vitamin C, raw multivitamin rich in trace minerals, gluten-free, raw diet rich with dark blueberries. 2T daily essential fatty acids like evening primrose oil or flax oil. Deep tissue lymphatic drainage on the extremities. Masai Barefoot Technology (MBT) shoes.

Obesity: Beet greens, celery, and parsley juiced daily. A raw diet for six months with the weekend juice fast each month. Colonics weekly or colon cleanse powder, 1 teaspoon daily.

Osteoporosis: Vitamins K and D. More dark greens and walking half an hour or more daily.

Parkinson's disease: Chlorella and more dark, leafy greens. Metals detox with EDTA, amino acids, and CoQ_{10}.

PMS: Evening primrose oil. Sea vegetables. Liver support teas like burdock or milk thistle. Juicing daily with lots of greens.

Psoriasis or *eczema:* Juice of carrots, celery, and lemon in the morning.

Rheumatoid arthritis: Juice of cucumber, endive, and dandelion. Nettle tea. 1 dried poke berry a day, orally. 2 T Borage oil daily. Eating a gluten-free vegan diet helps patients because RA is a systemic inflammatory disease that affects multiple joints of the body. A vegan diet is both atheroprotective and anti-inflammatory. Avoiding gluten is a must.

Teeth: Tooth oil made from raw coconut oil and tea tree or cinnamon has been used to prevent demineralization of tooth enamel. Recipe: 3 tablespoons (45 ml) coconut oil, 3 drops of tea tree or cinnamon essential oil. Stir. Put a few drops on your molars and brush into the rest of your teeth.

POSSIBLE EXCEPTIONS TO ORGANIC FRUITS AND VEGETABLES

In my recipes I suggest only organic fruits and vegetables. However, there are some foods that are reported to receive little if any pesticide contamination. Some people feel that these are safe to use:

- Avocados

- Oranges and grapefruit; other citrus fruits

- Coconuts (I suggest consuming young coconuts primarily)

- Watermelon

- Papayas (this is controversial, as some are now GMO)

- Mangoes

- Figs

- Garlic

- Some nuts, except peanuts

- Lavender (a fragrant herb often added to tea)

The Environmental Working Group has identified what it calls the "Dirty Dozen," the twelve most contaminated foods. Six of these are fruits, as noted in Table 14-1 on the following page.

TABLE 14-1	CONTAMINATED FRUITS AND VEGETABLES
Peaches	96 percent tested positive for pesticides
Strawberries	13 pesticides on a single sample
Apples	82 percent tested positive for pesticides
Blueberries	13 pesticides on a single sample
Nectarines	95 percent tested positive for pesticides
Imported grapes	Contaminated
Celery	13 different chemicals
Sweet bell peppers	61 percent tested positive for pesticides
Spinach	9 different chemicals
Kale	57 different chemicals
Collard greens	53 percent contaminated by pesticides
Potatoes	84 percent contaminated by pesticides

Washing these members of the "Dirty Dozen" in any solution does not remove pesticides or chemicals as the toxins are systemic, not just topical.

CHAPTER 15

Enzymes Prevent Premature Aging

*Disease stems from deficiencies and a lack of understanding of
Mother Nature's laws of health, plus the unwillingness to accept
the obligation to keep the precious temple—the body—in order.
This is accomplished by keeping it clean and well nourished.
And of course providing necessary aids—such as rest, relaxation,
positive thinking and plenty of exercise through hard work.*

—ANN WIGMORE, *WHY SUFFER: HOW I OVERCAME ILLNESS
AND PAIN NATURALLY*

Eating raw foods takes stress off an overworked endocrine system and aids the digestive system by adding enzymes that break down food. Enzymes are part of every metabolic activity. There are three major types of enzymes:

1. Enzymes that work in blood, organs, and our tissues, called metabolic enzymes.

2. Digestive enzymes.

3. Enzymes from raw foods.

If we eat too much processed food, we deplete the enzyme resources we are allotted at birth. The body that is starved of enzymes year after year ultimately will steal enzymes from enzyme-rich organs like the heart or pancreas. Enzymes keep us young and vital.

It is ironic that we have been brainwashed to believe that we need our RDA of beef, chicken, pork, milk, and dairy products. Why is so little advertising spent on the promotion of fresh fruits and vegetables?

I often tell students and patients that there is no true "aging process." What occurs is simply the depletion of enzymes and the subsequent loss of the body's ability to convert good, organic, biological food into energy. Vitality loss, immune collapse, disease, and degeneration always follow. The Standard American Diet leaves a person at a distinct disadvantage. If an athlete eats a boxed wheat cereal topped with milk and sugar for breakfast, fast food for lunch, and white flour pasta or a steak and potato for dinner, the body has not been fed what it needs to sustain a passive life, let alone an active one. In its infinite evolutionary wisdom, the body views running or running away as necessary survival activity. If enzymes to run are called for, the body will borrow enzymes from the heart. If you do this day after day—the body robbing Peter to pay Paul—the heart is eventually starved of enzymes. It's no wonder that we are hearing more news of runners who collapse and die due to heart failure. Technologically based medicine would have us believe that this malfunction stemmed from an unfortunate genetic predisposition. The runner was starved of enzymes and his body had none left to give. In the same manner, our bodies need to be fed vital nutrients, like magnesium and iodine. If our soils do not contain nutrients like iodine or magnesium in the first place, the plants cannot uptake them. We create a nutritional deficiency in our bodies that inhibits cellular transport, function, and repair. By the same token, we need enzymes to heal and to detoxify to remain young.

If we eat dead, cooked, denatured, processed foods on a regular basis, our body borrows enzymes for digestion and assimilation from the organs of the body itself. Two enzyme-rich organs are the pancreas and the heart, as I mentioned before. Eating cooked, enzyme-less food day after day forces our body to steal enzymes from the pancreas for digestive processes. The pancreas begins to swell, and eventually it is stressed into a disease process called type 2 diabetes. Research by Dr. Gabriel Cousens has proven that by eating a raw vegan diet on a daily basis for even a short time, the pancreas can probably begin to repair itself and the disease known as type 2 diabetes can possibly be reversed. If enzymes are not added to the diet and the pancreas is depleted of enzymes, the body, in its desire to continue the movement of life, will steal enzymes from the heart itself. The heart becomes stressed and enlarged due to the depletion of enzymes. Enzymes die in the cooking process if temperatures exceed 110–115 degrees Fahrenheit (43–46°C). Cooking also changes the biochemical structure of amino acids as proteins and fatty acids and renders them only partially digestible. Research has proven that you require less than half the amount of protein believed essential in the diet if the source of protein is raw in the form of leafy, green vegetables. In fact, these vegetables contain complete proteins of the highest quality. That is why eating four salad servings of leafy, green vegetables, such as romaine or red leaf lettuce, is a major consideration of this healing diet. Protein poisoning is a problem in this country. Protein poisoning can contribute to cancer and osteoporosis. There may be other considerations related to your particular health picture, including the health of the kidneys. If you need to eat less oxalic acid for any reason, it might be best to avoid the greens highest in oxalates, such as spinach or chard, or at least blanch them lightly for one to three minutes to leech our some of the oxalates. For the optimum healing diet, I recommend four servings of raw, organic leafy, green vegetables daily.

Because some fruits can be digested by the body in twenty minutes, part of my earlier training focused on fruits that could be eaten for breakfast or as a snack between meals. Some fruits do go well with other foods, so I encourage you to do more of your own research and experiment with living food recipes that allow you to mix them. I advise you to consume two servings of a variety of fruit daily. Fruit in season is by far the best. Do not eat the same fruit every day. However, if you have difficulty sleeping, it is beneficial to eat an apple after dinner and before bedtime. Apple pectin promotes the uptake of serotonin. It is generally best to eat fruit alone, but I do know many people who juice with apples or make blender drinks with leafy greens and various fruit choices. Listen to your body. For breakfast, we generally have a bowl of fruit with a few nuts that have been soaked in water overnight. Soaking the nuts makes them easier to digest and allows the nuts to release beneficial enzymes. Otherwise, we might drink a blended green smoothie that takes only minutes to create and keeps you feeling nutritionally satisfied until lunch.

CHAPTER 16

Outline of the 4-3-2-1 Raw Fasting Diet for Intensive Healing

It is interesting to know that I have never had a person come to me who was ill or in difficulty from eating too many fruits and vegetables; the trouble lies mainly with eating too many starches or animal proteins.

—BERNARD JENSEN, DC, PH.D., *BLENDING MAGIC*

Now we move on to the 4-3-2-1 three-month intensive healing diet. There is a reason for the ratio of 4-3-2-1: that is the maintenance of a proper alkaline pH. If you find that you are hungry, you might add up to two more servings of greens (from 4 to 6) and one more serving of cruciferous vegetables (from 3 to 4). This diet is pH-specific and will help you to heal faster if you are threatened by a disease. Refer to Chapter 11 concerning the benefits of raw juicing as well. I have patients who refer back to this diet and eat raw for three of the twelve months of the year to ensure wellness.

For three months, eat daily raw organic servings consisting of the following:

4–6 servings of leafy greens (use a variety, but no iceberg lettuce)

3–4 servings of varied cruciferous or starchy vegetables

2 servings of fruit (but only 1/2 banana at a time) and one apple daily

Note: Avoid fruit for the first two weeks if you have diabetes.

1 serving of nuts, grains, or seeds

Drink plenty of purified water daily. For example, if you are an adult who weighs 180 pounds (82 kg), you might consider drinking nine eight-ounce (227 g) glasses of water per day. Any type of herbal or green tea is also acceptable. I especially recommend alfalfa tea, which is good for healing the small intestine and reducing cholesterol, Pau D'Arco tea binds free yeast in the system, and ginger tea aids digestion if you do not suffer from elevated blood pressure. If you must drink coffee, please consume only one small cup of organic coffee in the morning.

See recipes at the end of this book that might enhance your RDA of vitamins and minerals and help you with meal planning. Diversity is a must. There are thousands of different types of produce. I encourage you to eat a rainbow of vegetables.

FOUR TO SIX LEAFY GREENS

Let's start with the largest group—the four to six servings of those leafy greens that I mentioned as natural detoxifiers. They are also an excellent source of bioavailable protein, vitamins, and minerals. Spinach, for example, contains more than twenty-three essential nutrients, including protein, iron, magnesium, calcium, vitamin K for the absorption of calcium, potassium, omega-3 fatty acids, sleep-assisting tryptophan, beta-carotene, folic acid, and vitamins C, B_1, B_2, B_3, and B_6. Kale, beet greens, and collard greens have many of the same nutrients, including the largest concentrations of sulfur-rich compounds, which allow the liver to produce enzymes that neutralize potentially toxic substances. Kale, collard greens, and spinach all also contain antioxidants that protect the lens of the eye. Collard greens, which make a great substitute for wraps in the diet, are one of the best plant-based sources of calcium. Romaine lettuce is an excellent source of chromium, which is an important mineral for blood sugar regulation. Romaine, like many other lettuce greens, contains folic acid, which protects the artery walls and prevents atherosclerosis. It also contains free radical–scavenging manganese. Two cups (400 ml) of romaine contains only sixteen calories. Most of the protein in leafy greens promotes muscle health. The different shades of leaf color in green leaves may not seem significant, but each shade represents a different combination of flavonoids and pigments that prevent disease. Quercetin is found primarily in green leaf salads, and this includes cilantro. For this reason, I encourage rotating or mixing leafy greens to ensure optimum health-promoting phytonutrients. Green salads promote cholesterol metabolism and a healthy heart. Four servings of greens daily will ensure that you have a greater chance of achieving an optimum alkaline pH balance of 7.5. Soaking the greens in cold water infused with organic vinegar for five minutes and then rinsing will help ensure that your food is residue- and dirt-free. Topping with a raw vegan dressing may further promote your health. I prefer an organic olive, sesame, or flax oil, blended with lemon juice, fresh herbs, garlic and Nama Shoyu, Bragg Aminos, or a wheat-free tamari. According to your particular health issue(s), you must decide which, if any, of those oils work for you. Vary your greens and eat them as frequently as you like throughout the day. If you find that you are hungry during the day, please eat more greens.

Several Leafy Green Vegetables

Arugula	Endive	Radicchio
Beet top greens	Escarole	Red Leaf
Butterhead or butter leaf	Frisée	Romaine
Cabbage (purple or green)	Kale	Spinach
	Mesculen mix	Sprouts
Chard	Lollo rosso	Watercress
Dandelion	Oak leaf	Young baby greens mix

MY FAVORITE LEAFY GREEN SALAD

Yield: Serves 2–4

Ingredients

3 kale leaves

1 chard leaf

1 cup (200 ml) baby spinach

1 cup (200 ml) mixed baby greens

1 stalk basil leaves, chopped

1 pressed clove of garlic in 4 tablespoons (60 ml) olive oil

2 tablespoons (30 ml) lime juice

2 tablespoons (30 ml) sesame oil

2 tablespoons (30 ml) Bragg Aminos

Pinch of natural sea salt

Directions

Roll kale leaves in sea salt to break down cell walls and digest more easily. Chop fine. Roll chard and then slice. Toss all other ingredients above and serve.

Variation: Add chopped celery, $^1/_2$ avocado, pine or other nuts, $^1/_2$ cup (200 ml) sprouts, 1 grated carrot

RED LEAF AND RASPBERRY SALAD

YIELD: SERVES 4

Ingredients

3 cups (600 ml) washed red leaf lettuce, torn to bite-sized pieces

$^1/_4$ cup (50 ml) fresh red raspberries, washed

$^1/_2$ Bosc pear, sliced thinly

6 tablespoons (90 ml) walnuts, pistachios, or pecans

1 tablespoon (15 ml) apple cider vinegar

$^1/_2$ teaspoon (3 ml) mustard

$^1/_2$ teaspoon (3 ml) salt

3 tablespoons (45 ml) olive oil

1 tablespoon (15 ml) toasted sesame (or plain) oil

Directions

Whip all but greens, fruit, and nuts in a bowl. Toss in remaining ingredients.

The Bitter Truth

You want me to eat dandelions? Yes. The French translation for *dandelion* is "tooth of the lion." Until you alkalinize and develop a taste for bitters in your raw diet, you may find the bitter taste of dandelion to be unpalatable. It may seem surprising that some people love the taste of fresh dandelions. It is speculated that there are differences in the taste buds of certain individuals that increase their ability to taste or not taste bitters. I feel that it has more to do with environmental food factors: if you grow up eating bitters, you seem to be able to munch them without wincing.

Many produce-conscious stores now sell these and other bitter greens, like arugula or frisée, with their salad selections. You can even wildcraft (pick where the soil has not been sprayed) young leaves prior to flowering from your yard. Bitters are an essential part of the human wellness picture because they thin the bile. A class of water-soluble phytochemicals, called sesquiterpenes, comprise the milky juice that makes a dandelion bitter. Rumor has it that shade-grown dandelion leaves contain fewer sesquiterpenes than those grown in direct sunlight. Bitters ensure proper digestion because they assist the gall-bladder and liver in thinning bile and in creating more digestive juices. To work, bitters should be experienced on the taste buds of the tongue, where the bitter taste is stimulated, saliva is secreted, and the gastric reflex causes digestive juices to be secreted. Food is better digested and assimilated because there is an increased flow of digestive juices from the pancreas, duodenum, and liver. Less undigested food is passed through the digestive tract. This relieves problems created by inefficient or allergy-antagonized digestion. I suggest that you introduce dandelion and other bitter greens to your diet slowly, a couple of leaves in your salad to start with until you can enjoy bitter greens as 25 percent of your salad.

MY DANDELION SALAD
YIELD: SERVES 4–6

Ingredients

About 10 leaves fresh dandelion greens, rinsed

$1/2$ head romaine or red leaf lettuce

$1/2$ cup (100 ml) red seedless grapes, sliced in half
(or 10 strawberries, sliced)

$1/2$ cup (100 ml) walnuts, sunflower seeds, or pecans, chopped

Directions

Cut or tear the greens into pieces. Mix all ingredients.

Variations: Add $1/4$ cup (50 ml) chopped red or green onions, or $1/2$ avocado, sliced.

DRESSING

Ingredients

1 tablespoon (15 ml) lemon juice

1 tablespoon (15 ml) agave nectar or raw honey

1 tablespoon (15 ml) almond butter or tahini

¼ cup (50 ml) olive oil

Optional: Kelp, sea salt, Bragg Aminos.

Directions

Whip all ingredients together. Add kelp, sea salt, or Bragg Aminos to taste.

THREE TO FOUR SERVINGS OF STARCHY VEGETABLES

Let's move on to the three to four servings of what I call fibrous, starchy, and cruciferous vegetables. All other vegetables that are not salad greens or leafy fit into this category, but red or green cabbage can fit into this category if you need it to. These should also be rotated and eaten throughout the day, so the body is presented with optimum nutrient combinations on a daily basis. I encourage you to make colorful choices. This would even include some of the starchier greens not on the salad inventory. I find it curious to learn that, in spite of a president's rejection of it, broccoli is one of the most popular green vegetables in the United States. Along with its other full complement of vitamins, minerals, and amino acids, broccoli contains a substance called indole-carbinol, which is reputed to prevent and slow tumor growth and prevent cancer cell metastasis. It also contains valuable nutrients that boost liver detoxification enzymes. Broccoli sprouts contain 10 to 100 times the power of mature broccoli to bolster enzymes and detoxify potential carcinogens. Brussels sprouts contain indoles that block the intercellular activity of estrogens that contribute to tumor growth and sulfur that prevents carcinogens from damaging healthy cells. The high fiber also contributes to colon cleansing, as do all of the fiber-rich vegetables. If you have a sluggish colon, Brussels sprouts may cause gas. Just keep in mind that this is part of the cleansing activity. I like to add Brussels sprouts to salads or make a salad combination from them by putting them in the food processor with garlic, olive oil, white balsamic vinegar, Bragg Aminos, and pine nuts. Add a tablespoon (15 ml) of hemp seed and/or sea vegetables as a salt or garnish.

Also in this category I include such tasty, healthy choices as the phosphorous-, fiber-, and foliate-rich legume sprouted lentils, plus red bell pepper, beets, cauliflower, sweet potatoes, carrots, peas, beans, onions, garlic, cucumbers, celery, squash, jicama, sea vegetables that are rich in minerals and iodine, fennel, radishes, and corn. While copper-rich olives and potassium- and fatty oleic acid–rich avocados are truly considered fruit, I would place their use as a food in this category. Research in 2005 found that adding avocados to salad or tomato increased the absorption of carotenoids in the bloodstream. I suggest that you use ground kelp or dulse instead of sea salt whenever possible while on this healing diet. Carrots, corn, sweet potatoes, and yellow squash are high in vitamin A carotenoids, which promote lung health. Carrots also contain bone-building vitamin K and phosphorus. Onions, leeks, and garlic are high in selenium and allicin, both of which promote a healthy heart and enhanced immune function. They, along with most cruciferous vegetables, also contain sulfur, a great detoxifier. Peas are high in B vitamins, which are essential for proper metabolism of fats, proteins, and carbohydrates. They also contain alpha- and beta-carotene. Fennel is rich in antioxidants as well as anti-inflammatory agents. It is delicious when combined with beets. Beets are known as powerful blood cleansers and, because they are very high in antioxidants, they are good for the heart. Celery contains coumarins, quercetin, and other nutrients that help to reduce blood pressure. Cauliflower has tryptophan, B vitamins, and muscle-building protein. Cauliflower is very low in saturated fat and cholesterol. It is also a good source of protein, thiamine, riboflavin, niacin, magnesium, and phosphorus, and it's a very good source of dietary fiber; vitamins C, K, and B_6; folic and pantothenic acid; potassium; and manganese. Cauliflower is a vegetable that is often ignored. As a member of the cruciferous family, it has many disease-fighting nutrients like indole-3-carbinol (13C) and sulforaphane. When Johns Hopkins University researched cauliflower, it found that sulforaphane lowered the occurrence of breast tumors in lab animals by 40 percent by sweeping out of the system toxins that normally damage cells and turn cancerous. The nutrient 13C with sulforaphane acts as an anti-estrogen that lowers the risk of tumor growth in the breast and prostate glands. Folate prevents anemia, cancer, and heart disease. Just four little florets of cauliflower a day will provide most of our daily vitamin C requirements.

Here is an overview of the various and numerous vegetables that you would certainly want to include in this category. Try to consume that awesome rainbow of colors in selecting your three daily servings from this group of vegetables that you eat throughout the day.

Cruciferous vegetables get their name from their cross-shaped (crucifer) flower petals. Research indicates that this family of vegetables may provide valuable cellular protection from certain types of cancers. This is due to indole-3-carbinol. This element changes the way that estrogen is metabolized and helps prevent estrogen-driven cancers. Also helpful in the prevention of cancer are the phytochemicals called isothiocyanates that stimulate our bodies to break down carcinogens. They are high in antioxidants like beta-carotene and the compound sulforaphane. They are rich in minerals, vitamins, and fiber.

The only concern regarding raw cruciferous vegetables is that they may contain thyroid inhibitors, known as goitrogens, that make it difficult for the thyroid to secrete its hormone. People with hypothyroid function should limit their consumption of goitrogenic, cruciferous raw vegetables or dip them in boiling water for sixty seconds, then immerse them in cold or icy water to prevent further enzyme damage.

Cruciferous Vegetables

Arugula	Chard	Mustard greens
Bok choy	Chinese cabbage	Radishes
Broccoli	Collard greens	Rutabagas
Brussels sprouts	Daikon	Turnips
Cabbage	Kale	Watercress
Cauliflower	Kohlrabi	

Other Starchy Vegetables

Beans, including green, white, pinto, garbanzo, limas	snap, black-eyed peas, purple hulled, split peas	Squash, including summer, winter, butternut, zucchini, and pumpkin.
Corn	Plantains	
Peas, including sugar	Potatoes	Sweet potatoes or yams

Some lists include beets and carrots, but these are also considered non-starchy.

Zucchini or Summer Squash Pasta

A company called Zyliss has a julienne peeler that creates thin, restaurant-style julienne strips (like pasta) with one easy stroke. You can use this when you peel a carrot, cucumber, or squash. In the same way, a spiral slicer or saladacco is a relatively low-tech gadget with a handle on top. This spins whimsical little discs out of squash or cucumbers on one side, and the other side of the blade creates pasta like strips. This allows you more flexibility in raw fooding, especially if you are a pasta lover. I'll share a couple of raw veggie pasta suggestions below.

RAW PASTA

Create julienne strips of summer or zucchini squash. Be certain to scrub or soak the outside skin with organic apple cider vinegar. Some people like to soak their pasta in ice water to firm it more, but I prefer to serve it immediately.

RAW SQUASH PASTA WITH TOMATO SAUCE
YIELD: SERVES 2

Ingredients

3 cups (600 ml) of raw squash "pasta"

1 large tomato, chopped

1 crushed garlic clove

½ teaspoon (3 ml) Italian herbs or 1 teaspoon (5 ml) each of thyme, oregano, and parsley fresh, chopped

¼ cup (50 ml) chopped basil

2 tablespoons (30 ml) olive oil

1 teaspoon (5 ml) Bragg Aminos or lemon

Variation: 6 sliced button or shitake mushrooms or sprinkle of 1 tablespoon (15 ml) nutritional yeast.

Directions

Stir together all sauce ingredients and pour over raw pasta.

RAW PASTA WITH PESTO SAUCE

*In the summer when we have lots of fresh basil,
I freeze fresh pesto from this recipe.*

YIELD: SERVES 2–4

Ingredients

3–4 cups (600–800 ml) raw pasta

2–3 cups (400–600 ml) fresh washed basil leaves

2–4 cloves of raw garlic

1 1/2 cups (300 ml) pine nuts, rinsed

1/4 cup (50 ml) olive oil

1/4 cup (50 ml) lemon juice

Sea salt (dulse or kelp may be used)
or dash of cayenne to taste

Directions

Blend all ingredients, except for the pasta. Pour over raw pasta. I refrigerate any leftover pesto to put on upcoming salads. It is delicious. (See also pistachio pesto for pasta topping in raw nuts, seeds, and grains.)

Variation: 1/2 avocado, added before blending

Add Cabbage and Kale to Your Raw Diet

There are over 400 varieties of cabbage. Three distinguishing types of cabbage families include stem, smooth leaf, and inflorescent:

- Stem cabbage includes kohlrabi, Chinese cabbage, kale, and collard greens

- Among smooth-leaf and curled-leaf cabbage are savoy, red, and green head cabbages

- Inflorescent cabbages include broccoli and cauliflower

Red or purple cabbage gets its color from the pigment anthocyanin. This is true of all red, blue, and purple plants. Red cabbage tends to be higher in fiber than green cabbage, but its leaves are also tougher. In a raw state, cabbage contains vitamin C, calcium, iron, and potassium. Red is higher than green in calcium, iron, and potassium. It is also higher in vitamins B_1, B_2, and B_3. Red can discolor if it is not fresh and shiny-looking, and it is sweeter if it is fresh.

There are lots of recipes for preparing cabbage, including using the fresh leaves as a wrap like burrito shells. When my intern, Dr. Jennifer Stanley, traveled to New Zealand to vacation and work on a kiwi farm, she discovered that they had lots of fresh red cabbage. She put her fantastic skills as a raw chef to good use and created great wraps for the entire crew. They loved them!

There are lots of creative variations of cole slaw, and it is an easy way to ensure your indole quota. Just shred any variety of cabbages or kale, or combine more than one variety for pretty texture and color. Add to your raw dish shredded carrots, a bit of lemon juice, olive oil, Bragg Aminos, and soaked, chopped nuts, such as walnuts, pine nuts, pecans, or Brazil nuts. You could even create a blender cashew olive oil and agave nectar topping.

One of my favorite ways to store and use shredded cabbage or chopped kale is to make "salted cabbage." You knead four cups (800 ml) of your choice in a tablespoon (15 ml) or more of sea salt and let it marinate and drain in a colander positioned over a bowl for about four hours. Rinse it and put it in a covered glass bowl in the refrigerator until you are ready to toss it in your salad. You can even use it in a layer with other shredded vegetables, such as broccoli or cauliflower or other leafy greens. It is nice to have this ready for travel or to add as a garnish. Having raw cabbage or kale on hand makes your diet more expansive: you can add chopped cabbage, kale, or collard greens to your blender or Vita Mix, along with other favorite vegetables and some water or juiced vegetables to make a raw soup. You can juice cabbage, kale, and collards; cabbage juice or raw, fermented cabbage juice (or sauerkraut juice) is a traditional drink to heal ulcers. In fact, in phytotherapy, cabbage is used to treat over one hundred illnesses. It stimulates the appetite and prevents scurvy. It kept Captain Cook's crew healthy. In one case, I feel that one product packaged in a jar might be an useful companion on your raw diet; it is raw sauerkraut or kim chi. Most health food stores carry both; just make certain the sauerkraut jar indicates "raw."

AVOCADO CABBAGE SALAD

Yield: Serves 2–4

Ingredients

$1/2$ green cabbage, cut into thirds and
processed into thin slices in a food processor

$1/2$–1 avocado, sliced into thin strips

$1/4$ sweet or red onion, sliced thin (use food processor)

2 tablespoons (30 ml) dill herb, dried or raw

2 tablespoons (30 ml) lemon juice organic,
or $1/4$ to $1/2$ raw lemon, squeezed

$1/2$ teaspoon (3 ml) dulse or kelp flakes (optional)

2 tablespoons (30 ml) olive oil

Directions

Mix all ingredients together lightly.

KALE SALAD

Yield: Serves 2–4

Ingredients

8 leaves of kale or 2 cups (400 ml), chopped fine

1 chopped or sliced avocado

1 raw tomato sliced, or $1/4$ cup (50 ml)
reconstituted sun-dried tomato

$1/4$ cup (50 ml) sweet or red onion, chopped

$1/4$ cup (50 ml) pine nuts, soaked for $1/2$ hour

1 garlic clove, crushed

$1/2$ teaspoon (3 ml) Italian spices

DRESSING

Ingredients

$\frac{1}{2}$ cup (100 ml) olive oil

1 tablespoon (15 ml) lemon juice

1 tablespoon (15 ml) Bragg Aminos

Directions

Mix all ingredients together lightly.

LEMON BROCCOLI

Just as the salt in salted cabbage softens the fiber, we like to add lemon to our chopped broccoli to soften it and make it easier to chew and digest.

YIELD: SERVES 2–4, DEPENDING ON SERVING SIZES

Ingredients

3 cups (600 ml) chopped broccoli florets

Juice of 1 fresh lemon

$\frac{1}{2}$ teaspoon (3 ml) sea salt

2 cloves fresh garlic

1 cup (200 ml) cilantro leaves

$\frac{1}{2}$ cup (100 ml) sunflower seeds,
cashews, or pine nuts.

1 teaspoon (5 ml) cumin seeds

$\frac{1}{4}$ cup (50 ml) olive oil

Directions

Stir the lemon and salt into the broccoli and let these three rest for about 40 minutes in the refrigerator. In the meantime, mince or press fresh garlic. Wash and chop cilantro leaves, then soak. Rinse and dry sunflower seeds, cashews, or pine nuts. Add garlic, cilantro, and seeds or nuts to the broccoli mix. Then add cumin seeds and olive oil. Mix well.

RAW "MASHED" POTATOES

One of my favorite recipes.

Ingredients

½ head raw cauliflower

Directions

In the food processor, process the cauliflower until it is smooth. If you like the texture more grainy, like rice, process it less.

Variation: You can add any spices you like, but my favorite is fresh or dried dill (2 teaspoons [10 ml]), a small clove of garlic or a dash of garlic powder, 6–8 tablespoons (90–120 ml) of olive oil, and a dash of sea salt.

TWO SERVINGS OF FRUIT

I recommend two servings of fruit daily. Because apples and apple pectin can help you absorb serotonin, you are able to get a better night's sleep, especially if you eat this apple as a snack sometime after dinner. Apples are also rich in fiber, which promotes good bowel function. I recommend the varieties that are less sweet and tend to be crunchy. Bananas are high in potassium, but because they, like oranges, are so sweet, I suggest that only one-half of either be eaten no more than three times a week on this healing diet. Please remember that bottled juices, like apple or orange juice, are not raw. Tomatoes, which are botanically classified as fruit, are high in cell-protecting antioxidants and lycopene, which are good for prostate health. Strawberries, peaches, grapes, blueberries, raspberries, blackberries, pineapple, papaya, apricots, and melons—all are excellent sources of antioxidants like vitamin C and natural anti-inflammatories. Blueberries are one of my favorite fruits, and they are high in resveratrol and flavonoids, which prevent free radical damage. Avocado, truly a fruit, is also rich in B vitamins and beneficial oils and contains all seven essential fatty acids, plus eighteen amino acids. Avocados are easily digested and contain more protein than cow's milk and more usable protein than a steak. In fact, all known enzymes are proteins, and of the twenty-two amino acids found in the body, eight must be derived directly from food. Vitamin C and beta-carotene are present in such wonder foods as raw oranges (do not drink bottled or frozen orange juice) and kiwi. In fact, kiwi has more vitamin C than oranges.

Many people who study a variety of raw fruits encounter an interesting character called the durian. I first heard of durian when my son returned from Thailand. He had a picture that he took near a bus stop that stated, "No Durian Allowed on Bus!" If you have never tried durian, you are missing an adventure. The smell is infamous and indescribable. My first taste of durian was at our first raw potluck. The durian owner had stored it in his garage since his wife would not allow it in the house. It tasted like pudding ambrosia, but smelled like dirty socks. I could only think that it was nature's way of protecting the fruit from those who might be tempted to consume it.

We eat only two servings of various fruits similar to the ones I mentioned above daily to keep insulin, blood sugar, and pH balanced. If you eat too many oranges or bananas during a week, you might develop a yeast overgrowth. If you have diabetes, it is best to avoid fruits or just occasionally eat a Granny Smith apple or avocado for the first month of this enzyme-rich diet.

Several Fruit Options

Apple: A global favorite fruit and a good source of vitamin C.

Apricot: Soft, sweet, and juicy orange-colored fruit packed with beta-carotene.

Avocado: Contains good fats, soft flesh, and a large stone in a thin outer peel. The trees produce hundreds of fruits, which taste buttery and rich. Peel to eat, or scoop out of the peel.

Breadfruit: A Malayan tree can produce up to two hundred or more grapefruit-sized fruits each season.

Banana: Yellow tropical fruit enjoyed the world over. In terms of sales, this tops the list of fruits.

Blackberry: Fruit of the bramble bush, which is a very common European wild bush. Blackberries are also cultivated, but the bush has sharp spines.

Blackcurrant: European native currant.

Blueberry: A North American fruit very high in nutritional antioxidants. The small bush grows in acidic soils, producing hundreds of small blue fruit in early summer.

Cherimoya, or custard apple: South American fruit, also grown in Hawaii, with white flesh that tastes of apples and custard. Seeds and skin are toxic.

Cherry: Related to both plums and apricots, the cherry tree produces small red fruit in midsummer.

Clementine: A sweet, orange, citrus fruit from the mandarin orange family. Clementines are much easier to peel than regular oranges.

Coconut: The fruit of the coconut palm is harvested throughout the tropical world for food and oil. In raw foods, we use young coconuts that appear white.

Cranberry: Also known as the American bog berry, cranberries are very high in vitamin C. Cranberries have an astringent taste and we use them dried in many raw recipes with walnuts and greens.

Dates: A nutritious and medicinal fruit of the date palm tree, generally dried and sweet. Dates contain fiber, sodium, protein, natural sugar, and vitamins A, C, E, and K, plus thiamine, riboflavin, niacin, B_6, B_{12}, folate, pantothenic acid, calcium, iron, magnesium, phosphorus, potassium, zinc, copper, manganese, selenium, plus saturated, monounsaturated, and polyunsaturated fat. Vitamin K, along with biotin and taurine, has been identified as one of the missing links to prevent osteoporosis.

The nicotinic content in dates prevents overgrowth of pathological organisms and aids the growth of beneficial bacteria in the intestines. Eastern studies have proven that soaked dates are beneficial for those who suffer from a weak heart. Dates have been used as a tonic for improving sexual stamina as well as some forms of reproductive problems. The soak water for dates has been used effectively against alcoholic intoxication. They are easily digested and supply quick energy.

Durian: A thorn-covered outer layer reveals a pudding-textured, strong-smelling fruit.

Fig: The fruit we know as the fig is actually the flower of the fig tree.

Grape: Clusters of white, yellow, purple, or red fruit that grows on vines in many parts of the world. Do not drink wine on this raw foods diet.

Grapefruit: Pink or white. Avoid it if you are on certain heart medications.

Guava: Round or oval fruit. Guavas are rich in vitamins A and C.

Jackfruit: Related to guava, but a much bigger fruit, which can grow to 80 pounds (36 kg). The taste is unusual. Popular in Asia.

Kiwi: Very high in antioxidants. Brown-skinned fruit with a hairy peel. Do not eat the peel, but scoop it out or pare it away. Great on salads or as a snack. Grown primarily in Australia, thus the name.

Lemon: The king of citrus fruits, lemon is tart and encourages the swallowing reflex.

Lime: A green relative of the lemon, but more bitter.

Loganberry: This tastes like a cross between raspberries and blackberries.

Mandarin: A type of orange that is smaller and easy to peel.

Mango: A tropical fruit that is very sweet and aids digestion.

Melon: There are many types of melon, including cantaloupe and honeydew.

Nectarine: A hairless type of peach. Peaches are more tender.

Orange: Popular citrus fruit with many different varieties.

Papaya: Many types of papaya. A great digestive aid and high in beta-carotene.

Peach: A favorite fruit of many Americans. Sweet inside and a bit hairy outside. I suggest peeling.

Pear: A northern European native that helps encourage gentle eliminations.

Persimmon: Also called *sharon fruit*. Persimmons are orange and must be seeded and peeled.

Pineapple: Very popular fruit, high in bromelain, a natural anti-inflammatory.

Plum: Small purple fruit that tastes sweet when ripe. The skin is sour.

Pomegranate: Red seedless or with seeds, pomegranates are juicy and fresh.

Strawberry: Use organic only. Sweet red, great on salads or as a dessert or snack.

Watermelon: A large melon with sweet, red, watery flesh. Very refreshing, especially in summer; good for kidneys, especially the seeds when used to make tea.

DATES IN YOUR WATER

Directions

Remove the seed and soak 3 dates overnight in $^1/_2$ cup (100 ml) purified water. Drink the water and eat the dates. May stir in crushed nuts and roll into cookies. Suggested use: as often as needed.

AVOCADO BOATS

YIELD: SERVES 3–4

Ingredients

2 or 3 ripe, pitted avocados

Fresh or frozen organic corn, $^3/_4$ cup (150 ml) or more

$^1/_2$ cup (100 ml) chopped cilantro leaves

1 or 2 tablespoons (15–30 ml) lime juice

1 crushed clove garlic

1 tablespoon (15 ml) olive oil

$^1/_4$ teaspoon (1 ml) cayenne powder

1 teaspoon (5 ml) sea salt

Directions

Cut avocadoes in half, score flesh into small squares, and spoon out avocado flesh. Remove the pit. Save the skins as "boats" to fill with mixture when finished.

Gently stir all ingredients together and refill avocado boats.

Variation: Top with raw salsa or chopped tomatoes.

Papayas, "Fruit of the Angels"

As a fruit, papayas are best eaten ripe to very ripe, as their antioxidant levels increase as they ripen. Papayas are a great source of antioxidants like vitamins C and A. Eating half a papaya, you receive twice the RDA of vitamin C and three-fourths of the RDA of vitamin A. Low in calories, they also contain nearly eighty other vital nutrients, including lycopene, folate, pantothenic acid, potassium, magnesium, and vitamins E and K. They are best eaten on their own, but occasionally we will juice papaya or use it in a blender smoothie. I have suggested dried papaya for patients who have difficulty digesting certain proteins because it contains the enzyme papain, which is extracted as a digestive dietary supplement known to prevent colon cancer. Papaya also inhibits oxidation of cholesterol. Oxidation allows cholesterol to stick to and build up in blood vessel walls, forming plaque, which can cause heart attacks or strokes. Papaya is also known for its anti-inflammatory effects, aiding asthma, osteoarthritis, and rheumatoid arthritis. It bolsters the immune system and inhibits macular degeneration. Research done at Kansas State University by Richard Baybutt indicates that vitamin A–rich foods promote lung health and can greatly reduce the effects of emphysema. Other research shows that lycopene may reduce a man's risk of developing prostate cancer. Other lycopene-rich fruits include tomatoes, apricots, pink grapefruit, watermelon, and guava. A tablespoon (15 ml) or more of papaya seeds may be blended in with raw salad dressing recipes and are useful in killing intestinal parasites.

ONE SERVING OF NUTS, SEEDS, GRAINS

In the final category, the *one* of the 4-3-2-1 healing diet, are the nuts, seeds, and grains. Just because they are last does not diminish their importance, especially when it comes to heart health. For example, almonds contain sixty vital nutrients, including vitamin E tocopherols and monosaturated fats that help prevent colon cancer, promote heart health and digestion, reduce body mass, and act like insulin medication in type 1 diabetics. The U.S. Food and Drug Administration considers almonds the king of nuts and suggests eating 1$1/2$ ounces (43 g) of almonds daily. Cashews, like walnuts, promote healthy joints. High in oxalates, they should be avoided if you have kidney challenges. Walnuts are high in omega-3 fatty acids and heart-healthy monosaturated fats. Walnuts and pumpkin seeds share a reputation as mild vermifuges, which kill intestinal parasites. For this reason, I suggest focused eating of these around the full moon when moon cycle parasites like tapeworms and roundworms awaken and reproduce. Like other seeds in this category, pumpkin seeds are high in zinc, muscle-relaxing magnesium, vitamin K, iron, protein, tryptophan, and copper. They build bone density and ensure joint health. Pumpkin seeds are so concentrated and so useful for muscle-building protein that they are considered one of the world's healthiest seeds. They also promote prostate health. Just one Brazil nut a day provides your RDA of selenium. Be sure to rinse all nuts and seeds in vinegar water and flush the tannins from the outside coverings. Then soak nuts overnight before eating them to enhance enzymes and aid digestion.

Sesame seeds are the first recorded seasoning, from 3000 BCE in Assyria. They are exceptionally high in calcium, far surpassing milk in that regard. One hundred grams (or 3 1/2 ounces) of sesame seeds contain 1,160 milligrams (mg) of calcium; a comparable amount of molasses contains 684 mg, while that same amount of milk contains only 130 mg of calcium. Research conducted by Dr. Deborah Sellmeyer and funded by a grant from the National Institutes of Health has proven that the animal proteins in dairy can contribute substantially to bone loss and weight gain. Her publication states: "Women with high animal to vegetable protein ratios were heavier and had higher intake of total protein. These women had a significantly increased rate of bone loss than those who ate just vegetable protein. Women consuming higher rates of animal protein had higher rates of bone loss and hip fractures by a factor of four times." Osteoporosis is *not* a problem that should be associated with lack of calcium intake. Americans get plenty of calcium daily. Osteoporosis results from calcium loss. "The massive amounts of protein in milk result in 50 percent loss of calcium in the urine. The calcium contained in leafy, green vegetables is more easily absorbed than the calcium in milk, and plant proteins do not result in loss the same way as animal proteins" (www.notmilk.com).

Besides calcium, sesame seeds are also rich in phosphorus, potassium, magnesium, iron, B_1, a lignin antioxidant, and vitamins E and A. Black sesame seeds are considered a kidney tonic, and in Oriental medicine, black sesame seeds are believed to prevent hair from graying. While there is a great deal of emphasis on calcium, magnesium is vital to enzymatic activity as well. It maintains proper pH in the body as well as ensuring proper absorption of calcium and neural and muscular (as in the heart) function. Without B_6 (pyridoxine) and magnesium, calcium phosphate stones accumulate, especially if you have daily intake of dairy products.

Nuts and seeds help to regulate blood sugar levels, and because they contain phytosterols or plant hormones, they also support the endocrine system and help to sustain sexual desire. They also prevent constipation and are excellent for bodybuilders or those who work with their muscles. Nuts and seeds are cholesterol-free and contain lipase, which controls fat and lowers LDL cholesterol levels in the body. Since soaking seeds activates protease and enzymes, I suggest soaking sesame seeds prior to making sesame milk. I am including Dr. Bernard Jensen's recipe for sesame milk, but I have also included another recipe from *The Raw Transformation,* by Wendy Rudell.

I believe that sesame seed milk is one of our best drinks.
It is a wonderful drink for lubricating the intestinal tract,
and its nutritional value is beyond compare as it is
high in protein, calcium, and other minerals.
—Bernard Jensen, DC, Ph.D., *The Chemistry of Man*

SESAME MILK: BERNARD JENSEN'S RECIPE

Directions

Blend in a blender for 1–$1/_2$ minutes $1/_4$ cup (50 ml) sesame seeds to 2 cups (400 ml) of pure water. Strain the liquid through a fine-wire mesh strainer or 2–4 layers of cheesecloth to remove hulls. You may add 1 tablespoon (15 ml) carob powder and 6–8 dates. For flavor or added nutritional value, any one of the following may be added to this drink: banana, raisins, apple, or cherry concentrate. Blend and strain. (I recommend adding a tablespoon [15 ml] of agave nectar and/or $1/_2$ teaspoon [3 ml] of vanilla to the original formula.)

Note: In place of sesame seeds, you could use almonds (nonirradiated and organic), pumpkin, or sunflower seeds, or a mix of all of them. It is best if you soak these nuts and seeds overnight to activate the enzymes.

SESAME MILK: WENDY RUDELL'S RECIPE

Directions

Add 1 cup (200 ml) soaked sesame seeds to 2–3 cups (400–600 ml) of purified water. Rinse seeds, blend, and strain. This is delicious over cereals or enjoyed by itself as milk. To sweeten, blend with dates, agave syrup, honey, or stevia. A wonderful substitute for dairy milk and superior in nutrients and enzymes.

Other uses for sesame seeds are in salad dressing, added to vegetable broth, added to fruits, mixed with nut butter, or for cereals for breakfast. Tahini, a paste like nut butters, is made from sesame seeds. Unhulled sesame seeds are high in oxalic acid, which can inhibit absorption of iron and calcium, while hulled seeds may be chemically treated and should be soaked overnight and rinsed to remove any residue.

Flax seeds and oil have been consumed since the time of ancient Greece. They are the most concentrated plant source of omega-3 fatty acids and alpha lipoic acid (ALA). They have anti-inflammatory properties as well as phytoestrogen lignans. I do not suggest peanuts as an option on this healing diet. Wild rice, actually a seed, can be prepared as an option. The grains in this category might include such giants as quinoa and amaranth. Fermented wheat, oat, and rye groats are often selected to make the probiotic-rich beverage rejeuvalac. The tiny grain quinoa must be rinsed thoroughly before sprouting to remove the naturally occurring pesticide that protects it from insects. Quinoa includes minerals and all nine essential amino acids. The lysine present in quinoa is essential for tissue and joint repair. Like amaranth and millet, quinoa sprouts overnight. Buckwheat is high in flavonoids, quercetin, the trace mineral manganese, and antioxidants.

Nuts

Almonds (buy only nonirradiated as raw)	Chestnuts	Pistachio nuts
	Filberts	Pumpkin seeds (these are truly seeds, but I list them here)
	Hazelnuts	
Brazil nuts	Hickory nuts	
Cashews (these are never sold raw because they are poisonous)	Macadamia nuts	Sunflower seeds (these, too, are truly seeds)
	Pecans	Walnuts

Edible Raw Seeds

Flax	Pumpkin	Sunflower
Hemp	Sesame	

Edible Raw Grains to Sprout

Amaranth	Lentils and mung (these are beans, but good to sprout)	Oat groats
Barley		Quinoa
Buckwheat		Wheat groats

How to Sprout Grains or Seeds

Note: How to best sprout seeds: Most seeds that are organic and untreated should sprout. Be sure that you store them in glass jars in a dark, cool area for safekeeping.

Basic Steps

1. Inspect and measure the appropriate amount of seeds and rinse them in vinegar water. Then rinse them in cool water until you are sure they are clean.

2. Put the seeds in a glass container or bowl and soak the seeds overnight in pure water that is at least double the amount of seeds.

3. Rinse the next day and drain off the water. Cover loosely and put in a 72-degree (22°C) oven or room temperature to ensure the sprouting process.

4. Rinse once a day until the sprouts show green leaves that are of optimum size for you. Note that at one point the sprouts look scruffy and need another day or two to sprout. The smaller the seed, the less time it takes to sprout. I sprout quinoa overnight only and rinse thoroughly before and after. Lentils take 4 days. Give your sprouts one final rinse in vinegar water and store them in the refrigerator or eat them as soon as possible.

EASY SPROUTED OATMEAL

Buy only whole organic oats, called "groats," not quick-rolled oats or flakes. Any good grocery or natural food store should carry them.

YIELD: SERVES 2

Ingredients

2 cups (400 ml) oat groats

6 pitted dates

2 cups (400 ml) water

2 tablespoons (30 ml) hemp seeds

1 teaspoon (5 ml) cinnamon

Dash of nutmeg

Directions

Rinse oat groats in vinegar water and soak in water overnight. Blend the oats, dates, and some water to make what looks like oatmeal consistency. Add hemp seeds, cinnamon, and nutmeg to taste.

Variations: You may add sesame or almond milk to cover the oatmeal cereal and sesame or flax oil to add to the sprouted oatmeal for more nutrition.

RAW PISTACHIO PESTO

Ingredients

1 1/4 cup (250 ml) fresh basil leaves

1 cup (200 ml) raw shelled pistachio nuts

1/2 cup (100 ml) cilantro

3 cloves garlic

2/3 cup (132 ml) olive oil or more

1 teaspoon (5 ml) lime or lemon zest

1 teaspoon (5 ml) Bragg Aminos or 1/2 teaspoon (3 ml) sea salt

1 tablespoon (15 ml) nutritional yeast (optional)

Directions

Pulse all ingredients in the food processor or blender and purée until smooth. Use as raw pasta topping or fill celery or red pepper strips with pesto. Freezes well.

TRAVELING TABOULI (QUINOA OR LENTIL SPROUTS)

This recipe is great to take along anywhere, even on airplanes!

Ingredients

1 cup (200 ml) sprouted quinoa or lentils

1/2 cup (100 ml) chopped tomato

¼ cup (50 ml) chopped cilantro

¼ cup (50 ml) pine nuts or pecans

1 stalk chopped celery

1 tablespoon (15 ml) lemon juice fresh

2 tablespoons (30 ml) olive oil

1 tablespoon (15 ml) chopped mint or dill

1 tablespoon (15 ml) Bragg Aminos

Directions

Toss all ingredients and place the mixture in a glass or recyclable container. Refrigerate.

Variation: Add chopped green onions. You could even mix quinoa or lentils together and add chopped avocado.

RAW YUMMY CHILI

YIELD: SERVES 4–6

Ingredients

1 cup (200 ml) sprouted lentils

1 portobello or 6 button mushrooms, chopped

¼ cup (50 ml) chopped onion

½ red bell pepper, chopped

2 cloves fresh garlic

½ cup (100 ml) almonds or pecans,
soaked overnight

1 stalk celery, chopped fine

2 cups (400 ml) chopped tomatoes
or 1 cup (200 ml) sun-dried tomatoes

1 tablespoon (15 ml) each: cumin, oregano,
agave nectar, apple cider vinegar, olive oil

1 teaspoon (5 ml) chili powder

¼ teaspoon (1 ml) cayenne

⅛ cup (25 ml) Bragg Aminos

Directions

If you're using sun-dried tomatoes, soak the tomatoes in 2 cups (400 ml) of water and blend tomatoes and water, garlic, spices, and nuts. You may either gently pulse in the rest of the ingredients to the desired consistency, or just pour the tomato blend over the other ingredients. Add sea salt to your taste. Serve at room temperature or store in refrigerator.

Variations: This recipe can be made with a blend of sun-dried tomatoes and fresh chopped tomatoes.

The ANDI Score for Beans, Nuts, Grains, and Seeds

ANDI is the acronym for "Aggregate Nutrient Density Index." The ANDI (sometimes called MANDI) score was designed by Dr. Joel Fuhrman to guide consumers to optimum micronutrient- and vitamin-dense foods. The goal is to achieve a score of 100 points per day. It is an interesting evaluation, and one you might consider for your meals, per cup serving below.

Beans

Lentils (104)	Adzuki beans (84)	Edamame (58)
Red kidney beans (100)	Black beans (83)	Split peas (58)
Great northern beans (94)	Black-eyed peas (82)	Chickpeas/garbanzo beans (57)
	Pinto beans (61)	

Nuts and Seeds

Sunflower seeds (78)	Pistachios (48)	Walnuts (34)
Sesame seeds (65)	Pecans (41)	Hazelnuts (32)
Flax seeds (65)	Almonds (38)	Cashews (27)
Pumpkin seeds (52)		

Whole Grains

Oats, old-fashioned (53)	Barley, pearled (32)	Quinoa (21)
Barley, whole-grain (43)	Wheat berries (25)	Millet (19)
Wild brown rice (43)	Cornmeal, whole-grain (22)	Bulgar (17)
Brown rice (41)		

CHAPTER 17

The Miracle of Sea Vegetables: Nutrient-Dense Iodine and Trace Minerals

It's often said that you are what you eat.
I say that you are what you absorb.
—BERNARD JENSEN, DC, PH.D.,
THE SCIENCE AND PRACTICE OF IRIDOLOGY, VOL. 1

I always get a blank stare when I encourage patients to add sea vegetables to their diet. Why would anyone want to eat sea vegetables? Nutrient-dense sea vegetables offer the widest range of minerals of any food, containing all the minerals found in the ocean. These same minerals mimic the constitution of human blood. Without minerals, vitamins cannot be used by the body. Sea vegetables are an amazing source of iodine and vitamin K. They are a very good source of the B-vitamin folate and magnesium, as well as a good source of iron and calcium. Also present are the B-vitamins riboflavin and pantothenic acid. Sea vegetables contain lignans, which are plant compounds with cancer-protective and tumor-inhibiting properties. Sea vegetables (especially kelp) are nature's most abundant source of iodine, which as a component of the thyroid hormones known as thyroxine, T4, and triiodothyronine, T3, is essential for human life. The thyroid gland adds iodine to the amino acid tyrosine to create T3 and T4. Without sufficient iodine, your body is not able to synthesize them. Thyroid hormones regulate metabolism in every cell of the body. In addition, they are involved in nearly all physiological functions. Since this is the case, an iodine deficiency can have a devastating effect on your health and well-being. A common sign of thyroid deficiency is a goiter, an enlarged thyroid gland. Folic acid in sea vegetables has a number of other very important protective functions. Appropriate levels of folic acid in the diet are needed to prevent certain birth defects, including spina bifida. Folic acid also breaks down a dangerous chemical produced during the methylation cycle called homocysteine. Homocysteine can damage blood vessel walls and increase the risk of cardiovascular disease and stroke. The magnesium present in sea vegetables makes them a heart-effective addition to salads and raw soups daily.

Fucans present in some sea vegetables have been shown to reduce the body's inflammatory response, while the magnesium present acts as a natural relaxant to help prevent migraine headaches and reduce the severity of most asthma symptoms.

Sea vegetables' relaxing magnesium may also promote normal sleep for women who are experiencing symptoms of menopause, while the lignans may act as very weak versions of estrogen that alleviate the discomfort of hot flashes.

Where do sea vegetables come from? They grow in marine saltwater as well as in freshwater lakes. Sea vegetables depend on some sunlight penetrating the water, yet they are not plants or animals—they are actually algae. They are classified into categories by colors: red, brown, or green. They all have a unique taste, texture, and shape, and I suggest that if you do not like one type of seaweed you try its cousin. Nori is probably the best known in America, when it comes to sushi fans. Raw nori is best for a raw diet, but some choose toasted nori. It is the dark, nearly black wrapper around the roll. Kelp and dulse flakes or strips are easy to find in most Asian groceries or health food stores. Kelp is brownish green, and dulse a reddish brown color. I suggest that you put these in the spice grinder and use them instead of salt on salads or in raw vegetable soups. Wakame, kombu, arame, and hijiki (use the organic versions only) are often added to miso soup. While miso is not a raw product, it is fermented, and I find that many raw patients in the Midwest appreciate adding it occasionally to their diet in the cold of winter.

Japan is the largest producer and exporter of sea vegetables, and that explains their Oriental names. If you can purchase organic sea vegetables, you run less risk of any potential mercury or arsenic contamination. The rich mineral content and its reputation for being a detoxifier itself make sea vegetables among the world's healthiest foods.

SIX WAYS TO USE SEA VEGETABLES

1. Use nori as a wrap for sprouts, avocado, and nut patés.

2. Add nori, dulse, or kelp to smoothies, raw soups, or salads.

3. Use as a Gomashio condiment (see recipe on page 203).

4. Make a seaweed slush and use it as a dip or add it to drinks or dressings (see recipe on page 204). Add strained seaweed slush to juice when fasting.

5. Use kelp or dulse flakes or powder instead of sea salt in any recipe.

6. Use seaweed paste on your face as a mask or in your tub as a soak.

RAGING IODINE DEFICIENCY IN THE UNITED STATES

The body produces no iodine, and the thyroid is the only organ that can store large quantities of iodine. In most areas of America, the soil has always contained very low levels of iodine. Because of over farming and poor farming practices, iodine is no longer present in our soils. If iodine is not present in the soil, our plants cannot absorb it as a nutrient or manufacture it. For that reason, we no longer get adequate iodine from the plants we consume. To compensate for this, food manufacturers in the past attempted to add iodine to chemically created salt, bread, and milk. Because it adds additional cost, iodine is no longer added to bread or milk. People believe that iodine in salt is sufficient, but the amount of iodine added to salt has declined over the years. It is no wonder there is a plague of iodine deficiency in the United States.

Health problems come with iodine deficiency. Iodine has natural antimicrobial, antibacterial, and antifungal properties. Research shows that iodine deficiency in the thyroid causes the thyroid to become enlarged and then manifests as a thyroid goiter. There is also a high incidence of thyroid cancer in countries where iodine is not in the diet at all. Most people over age sixty are encouraged to reduce their salt intake because of high blood pressure. As a result, they become depleted of iodine because of lack of iodine in their diet. This age group has the highest occurrence of thyroid nodules and goiters. Nearly a quarter of people in this age category will become senile as a result of low iodine or hypothyroidism. Iodine supplementation or eating Japanese seaweed may alleviate these iodine-related diseases.

Iodine is concentrated in the glandular system, even the body's sweat glands. The ovaries, breasts, prostate, and brain contain high concentrations of iodine. Nearly every cell in the body is dependent on this important element. When a deficiency of iodine occurs, the thyroid competes with other storage sites and all of them then become depleted. A continued deficiency puts a person at risk for a variety of conditions and illnesses.

Iodine is concentrated in breast tissue, and a lack of iodine in the breasts creates fibrocystic breast disease. This may lead to cystic breasts that engorge prior to the menstrual period and become quite painful. It is estimated that over 95 percent of American women have fibrocystic breast disease. The longer this disease exists in the body, the higher the risk for developing of breast cancer. Since some 20 percent of all iodine in the human body is stored in the sweat glands of the skin, lack of iodine manifests as dry skin with a decreased ability to sweat.

Insufficient iodine in the stomach can cause inadequate digestive acid production, a condition known as achlorhydria. Iodine is used by the stomach's parietal cells to concentrate chloride, which is used to produce hydrochloric acid for digestion. With the prolonged lack of hydrochloric acid, a person has a much higher risk of developing opportunistic *Helicobacter pylori (H. pylori)* or even stomach cancer.

A lack of iodine can cause dry eyes, since iodine is concentrated in the lachrymal glands. Similarly, dry mouth may be caused by a deficiency of iodine. Iodine is concentrated in the glands of the mouth, and if there is an iodine deficiency, this can result in dry mouth.

Iodine deficiency can cause cysts to grow in the ovaries, called polycystic ovary disease (PCOS). The greater the iodine deficiency, the more ovarian cysts a woman produces. In Japan, the Japanese population consumes approximately 13.8 mg of iodine a day from seaweed specifically cultured to maximize iodine. The Japanese have the lowest incidence of female reproductive organ cancer in the world. It is also crucial for women of reproductive age and those nursing babies to have sufficient iodine. Iodine is very important in the first three years of development of life: for the fetus growing inside the womb until two years following birth. The World Health Organization has reported that a deficiency of iodine is the primary cause of preventable mental retardation and brain damage in infants. A child's IQ can be enhanced by iodine, so it is beneficial to consume adequate Japanese seaweed during pregnancy and for two years while nursing.

David Brownstein, M.D., explains in his book, *Iodine: Why You Need It, Why You Can't Live Without It,* how the thyroid requires iodine to produce hormones and regulate the body's metabolism. Hypothyroidism is indicated by a low metabolic rate, and symptoms include cold hands and feet, poor memory, elevated cholesterol, fatigue, inability to concentrate, infertility, menstrual problems, muscle cramps, weight gain, puffy eyes, and brittle fingernails. Eating seaweed or taking an iodine supplement under the supervision of a health care professional can help to cure or alleviate these issues as symptoms as well as address the underlying root cause of hypothyroidism.

We must also consider another issue related to our toxic environment. Exposure to toxic chemicals known as halides (bromide, fluoride, chloride, and iodide) hinders the absorption of iodine in the body. Iodide is the only halide with therapeutic effects in the body. These xenotoxins act as endocrine disruptors and compete for iodine receptor sites. Unfortunately, in the 1980s, bromine, a known breast carcinogen, replaced iodine as a bread dough ingredient. This FDA-approved change by the food industry resulted in an epidemic of bromide toxicity and increases in thyroid disorders, thyroid cancer, and other illnesses stemming from iodine deficiency. Bromine, which is also approved for crop fumigation and pest control, is present in some carbonated drinks and several prescription medications as well.

Exposure to chlorine and fluoride found in toothpaste, the water supply, and many pharmaceutical drugs further adds to iodine deficiency because these toxins compete with iodine for absorption by body tissues. If you have sufficient iodine saturation in bodily tissues, this prevents the binding of halides and allows for their elimination from the body.

Dr. Brownstein tested for iodine sufficiency in more than 4,000 patients and found 96 percent of them to be deficient. Dr. Jorge Flechas has had similar results in lab tests of more that 21,000 cases worldwide. It is useful to consider that the mainland Japanese ingest nearly 14 mg of iodine daily from enriched seaweed, and that is almost 100 times more that the U.S. Recommended Daily Allowance. These are considered extreme amounts by U.S. standards, yet the Japanese have very low rates of endocrine disorders as compared to Americans. These include fibrocystic breast disease, as well as breast, endometrial, ovarian, and prostrate cancers. We should consume Japanese seaweed daily.

DR. MITCHELL'S
RAW GOMASHIO RECIPE

I learned a version of this recipe (see toasted recipe below) nearly thirty years ago when I was studying macrobiotic cooking. The only difference is that now I often make it raw. If it is raw, keep it in the refrigerator and it should last for a month or so. We add Gomashio to our vegetables and salads.

Ingredients

1 cup (200 ml) raw organic white or black sesame seeds

1 or 2 teaspoons (5–10 ml) of kelp or dulse powder
(2 teaspoons [10 ml] if no sea salt is added)

1 teaspoon (5 ml) gray sea salt (optional)

Directions

Grind all ingredients together in spice grinder and store.

DR. MITCHELL'S
TOASTED SEAWEED GOMASHIO

Ingredients

14 ounces (397 g) freshly ground sesame seeds
(grind in a spice grinder)

1 ounce (28 g) ground kelp, dulse, or wakame

1 ounce (28 g) real or gray sea salt

Directions

Fry all the ingredients in a dry skillet until the ground sesame appears toasted.

Use as condiment daily.

DR. MITCHELL'S
SEAWEED SLUSH

Directions

Cover and soak 1 package of kombu in purified water for 4 hours. Blend and store. Use in salad dressings, soups, and smoothies. You may also purify and drink this slush or use it (strained) in enemas. Add 1 tablespoon (15 ml) honey and put it on your face as mask. Leave it on for fifteen minutes or more.

DR. MITCHELL'S
SEAWEED PURÉE

Directions

Strain seaweed "slush" of water and add 1 cup (200 ml) of sesame or olive oil. Blend and add to salad dressing recipes, wherever you would use olive oil in a recipe. You might use seaweed purée to obtain more nutrients.

ORGANIC HIJIKI WITH CARROTS,
ONIONS, AND GOMASHIO

Hijiki is a fine-filament dark seaweed used frequently in Japanese cooking.

Ingredients

2 cups (400 ml) dried hijiki,
soaked for 10 minutes, then drained

½ cup (100 ml) onions, chopped very fine

4 large carrots, grated or julienned

1 tablespoon (15 ml) sesame oil

1 teaspoon of Bragg Aminos

Directions

Blend all ingredients and garnish with Gomashio.

WAKO SALAD: WAKAME, AVOCADO, KALE, AND ONIONS

Ingredients

1 cup (200 ml) wakame, soaked 4 hours, drained, and chopped

8 leaves of kale, rolled continuously in $1/2$ teaspoon (3 ml) salt until fibers are soft; rinse and chop

1 diced large avocado

2 green onions, finely chopped

1 tablespoon (15 ml) toasted sesame oil

$1\frac{1}{2}$ tablespoons (23 ml) Bragg Aminos

$1\frac{1}{2}$ tablespoons (23 ml) brown rice vinegar

Directions

Stir all ingredients and marinate the mixture in the refrigerator for several hours. Garnish with Gomashio or toasted or raw sesame seeds just before serving.

NORI ROLLS OR NORI SALAD

Ingredients

2 cups (400 ml) raw nuts, like almond, walnuts, or pecans, soaked in 1 tablespoon (15 ml) brown rice vinegar

2 diced avocados

2 shredded carrots

2 diced cucumbers (cut in 2 and rub cut ends together to remove bitterness)

2 sliced red peppers

2 tablespoons (30 ml) Bragg Aminos

2 tablespoons (30 ml) toasted sesame oil

Nori seaweed sheets

Directions

Mix finely chopped nuts with rice vinegar. Add vegetables and mix. Add Bragg Aminos and sesame oil. Fold nori and cut into small strips. Mix into the salad or put vegetable and nut mixture onto nori and roll into sushi rolls just before serving. Cut into 1–2-inch (2.5–5 cm) pieces with a sharp, serrated knife.

WAKAME CUCUMBER SALAD

Ingredients

2 cucumbers, chopped (cut in half and rub cut ends together to remove bitter taste; rinse)

2 red peppers, finely chopped

1 red onion, finely chopped

2 medium tomatoes, chopped

2 cups (400 ml) wakame seaweed, soaked, then drained and chopped

2 tablespoons (30 ml) brown rice vinegar

1 1/2 tablespoons (23 ml) Bragg Aminos

2 tablespoons (30 ml) raw honey

2 tablespoons (30 ml) toasted sesame oil

Directions

Mix brown rice vinegar, honey, and sesame oil. Stir into the vegetables and seaweed.

SEA VEGETABLE SOUP: "BIRTHDAY SOUP"

Birthday Soup is often given to mothers in Japan recovering from childbirth. It is easy to digest and high in iron, calcium, protein, iodine, and other minerals. I have included mushrooms in the recipe to add zinc to the soup.

Ingredients

1 ounce (28 g) wakame, dulse, or nori seaweed,
soaked in 1 cup (200 ml) hot water (reserve for later)

4 button or shitake mushrooms, cleaned and chopped

1 tablespoon (15 ml) sesame oil

2 cloves of garlic, chopped or sliced

2 tablespoons (30 ml) Bragg Aminos

1 teaspoon (5 ml) each basil and thyme

Directions

Blend all but the mushrooms in the recipe above. You may also add 1 tablespoon (15 ml) of organic miso if you choose, as well as raw coconut milk. Add mushrooms as a garnish or blend if you want the soup to be smooth.

SEA VEGETABLE TAPENADE

Ingredients

$1/3$ cup (66 ml) dulse or kelp flakes

5 cloves of garlic, crushed

$1/4$ cup (50 ml) extra-virgin olive oil

1 cup (200 ml) kalamata olives, chopped

Directions

Pulse all ingredients in a food processor. Makes a great dip for all vegetables or a dressing on romaine.

CHLORELLA: FRESHWATER ALGA

Hair Mineral Testing for Biohazardous Materials

Whenever I do a hair mineral analysis test, I am amazed at the biohazards found in the human body. Diseases that may result from heavy metal poisoning include heart disease, cancer, diabetes, depression, anxiety, infections, autism, chronic fatigue, chemical sensitivities, autoimmune disorders, and many other conditions. Heavy metal detoxification is possible through nutritional therapy, which involves reversing disease processes by binding and removing the toxic metals and then replacing them with the preferred vital minerals. Most biological naturopaths are adept at detoxification and will offer remedies to alleviate many physical, mental, emotional, and behavioral health conditions, including chronic diseases. Hair mineral analysis is an inexpensive and accurate tool used to assess abnormalities not detected through other routine tests. However, most insurance companies will not pay the modest laboratory fee because it is considered a "crime lab" test. Hair analysis provides information about metabolism on the cellular level. It assesses glucose tolerance, organ and glandular function, energy level, metabolic rate, and disease susceptibility based on the state of the immune system. Hair mineral analysis is also a powerful tool to identify biochemical causes of mental, emotional, and behavioral conditions. Minerals control neurotransmitters and other neuroactive chemicals, but all the toxic metals are neurotoxic and have a profound negative effect on the brain. Depression, anxiety, epilepsy, phobias, insomnia, fatigue, mood swings, attention-deficit disorder, and learning disorders may all be a result of neurotoxic chemicals. Additionally, the hair mineral analysis gives naturopaths an indication of which type of nutritional therapy or detoxification to employ as well as a guide for monitoring progress. Comparing the results of mineral tests over a period of months is a way to monitor subtle changes in body chemistry. Only about one teaspoon (5 ml) of hair is required from the nape of the neck.

Toxic elements that are tested include aluminum, antimony (used as a waterproof ingredient in mascara and eyeliner as well as a flame retardant), arsenic, barium (a byproduct of the battery industry and other industries, whose plants dumped it in agricultural areas to dispose of it), bismuth (present in many stomach-soothing products), and cadmium (from many sources, including tap water, fungicides, marijuana, processed meat, rubber, seafood [such as cod, haddock, oysters, and tuna], sewage, tobacco, colas from vending machines, tools, welding material, evaporated milk, airborne industrial contaminants, batteries, instant coffee, incineration of tires or rubber or plastic, refined grains, softened water, galvanized pipes, dental alloys, candy, ceramics, electroplating, fertilizers, paints, motor oil, and motor exhaust). Excess cadmium is associated with the following diseases: alopecia (hair loss), anemia, arthritis, cancer, lung disease, cerebral hemorrhage, cirrhosis of the liver, enlarged heart, diabetes, emphysema, hypoglycemia, hypertension, impotence, infertility, kidney disease, learning disorders, migraines, inflammation, kidney disease, osteoporosis, schizophrenia, strokes, vascular disease, elevated LDL cholesterol, impaired growth, and cardiovascular disease. You may feel lethargic because cadmium inhibits essential enzymes in the Krebs energy cycle, where a compound called adenosine triphosphate (ATP) provides cells with the energy needed for life. Cadmium can directly damage nerve cells and underlie a tendency for hyperactivity of the nervous system. Toxic levels of cadmium can contribute to arthritis, osteoporosis, and neuromuscular diseases. Cadmium may make arteries brittle and inflexible. It accumulates in the kidneys, resulting in high blood pressure and kidney disease. Cadmium toxicity can alter calcium and vitamin D activity and cause extreme restlessness and irritability, headache, chest pain, increased salivation, choking, vomiting, abdominal pain, diarrhea, throat dryness, cough, and pneumonia. Cadmium as a toxin can cause asthma and emphysema because the cadmium is antagonistic to the enzymes in the main lung alveoli.

Then we come to the toxic elements of lead, mercury, and nickel. These toxic three are or were used in various forms and ways in vaccines, mercury amalgam dental fillings, and contact lens solutions. Thallium, tin, and uranium are extremely toxic. Thallium causes anxiety, nervous tendencies, alterations in the spinal cord, and alopecia (hair loss). Tin causes headaches, vomiting, diarrhea, abdominal cramping, abdominal bloating, nausea, fever, hyperglycemia, vision changes, and liver pain. Excess tin accumulates in the brain and can cause brain damage and severe headaches. It can also accumulate in the liver and cause liver damage. Tin can also irritate the gastrointestinal tract and cause vomiting and diarrhea. Mercury and nickel can cause severe sleep disturbances.

What is shocking to me is the amount of uranium, mercury, aluminum, antimony, lead, and nickel that I am finding in Midwestern children and adults. Remember the Stanford cord-blood studies? Babies are born with, on average, over two hundred toxic substances in their blood! Excessive toxic metals from our polluted environment and foods, such as mercury or cadmium, may accumulate in the body due to chronic exposure and may lead to metal toxicity illnesses. Many illnesses develop as people are exposed to high levels of heavy metal toxicity, which depress the immune system and allow diseases to enter the body. When mineral deficiencies occur, toxic metals replace the missing essential minerals in enzyme-binding sites. This allows the body, in its innate intelligence, to survive in the face of nutrient deficiencies. These elements may inhibit enzymes in your body, weaken cell membranes, or impair nutrient delivery, which can lead to metal toxicity illness. Exposure most commonly occurs through everyday living, but may result from an industrial work environment; other means are exposure to cigarette smoke (cadmium), hydrogenated oils (nickel), antiperspirants or antacids (aluminum, yes—it is still there regardless of what you've been told), some toothpastes and cans (tin), tap water (lead), and dental fillings and fish (mercury).

Heavy metal toxicity in children may be related to the following symptoms: decreased intelligence, immune dysfunction, nervous system disorders, fatigue, depression, memory loss, diarrhea, skin rashes, anemia, muscle pain or weakness, nausea, irritability, tremors, behavioral problems including hyperactivity, autism, cancer, or headaches.

The good news is that heavy metal detoxification is possible through nutritional therapy, which involves reversing disease processes by replacing the toxic metals with the preferred vital minerals. So if you or your loved ones suffer from allergies; high blood pressure; gastrointestinal issues including bloating, diarrhea, and gas; mood swings; difficulties with concentration or memory retention; infections; poor night vision; wounds healing slowly; periodontal symptoms; poor taste or smell (both are altered by aging, but aging reflects an accumulation of metals); or skin conditions, I would ask your naturopath to perform a hair mineral analysis to see what toxic elements may be harming your health.

GOOD NUTRIENTS

Your nutritious minerals are tested in the hair mineral analysis. Those good elements are boron, calcium, chromium, cobalt, copper, iron, lithium, magnesium, manganese, molybdenum, phosphorus, rubidium, strontium, sulfur, vanadium, and zinc. Genova Diagnostics Laboratory in Ashville, North Carolina, has provided research that indicates how low levels of these minerals may be associated with some of the following disease processes:

Low zinc is associated with poor wound healing, weight problems, depressed libido, hair loss, acne, anorexia, body odor, benign prostate hyperplasia, and impotence.

Low manganese is associated with back and joint problems, hypoglycemia, and allergies.

Low selenium is associated with age spots.

Low calcium, chromium, and vanadium may contribute to attention deficit disorder.

Low calcium, magnesium, molybdenum, and selenium may contribute to cancer.

Low chromium, molybdenum, selenium, and zinc are associated with candida.

Low chromium (may contribute to bipolar disorder) and sulfur are associated with anxiety.

Low boron, calcium, copper, sulfur, and zinc are associated with arthritis.

Low calcium, magnesium, manganese, molybdenum, potassium, sulfur, and zinc are associated with asthma.

Low molybdenum is associated with environmental allergies, bladder infections, canker sores, and athlete's foot.

Low cobalt may be associated with myelin sheath damage.

And there are hundreds more.

While copper is a good element, if it is out of balance, it can cause disastrous results. According to the Genova Diagnostics Lab:

> Doctors at Loyola University Medical School in Chicago and the Carl Pfeiffer Treatment Center have reported that violent males between the ages of 3 and 18 commonly have elevated copper and reduced zinc blood levels when compared to nonviolent males. Depression and schizophrenia also have links to high copper levels; also cirrhosis of the liver, hepatitis, mental disorders, headaches, premature hair loss and breast cancer. Element imbalances are linked to: fatigue, headaches, osteoporosis, malnutrition, depression, hypoglycemia, cancer, aggressive behavior, allergies, joint pain, diabetes, digestive disorders, learning disabilities, attention deficit disorder, autism, and hypothyroidism. Without minerals, vitamins have absolutely no function in the body. The key factor to reversing disease, including heavy metal detoxification, is maintaining a balanced acid-alkaline state in the body. As a general rule, acid substances tighten; and alkaline substances relax. Minerals are alkaline because they relax the body from tightness, tension, stiffness, spasms, twitches, tics or jerkiness as in nervousness, anxiety, anger, fear, agitation, headaches, muscle cramps, menstrual cramps, arthritis, insomnia, constipation, heart palpitations, irregular heartbeats, high blood pressure, eye twitches, acne, plaque on teeth, plaque on heart and arteries due to cholesterol build-up,

plaque on the brain [Alzheimer's], and an accumulation of estrogen build-ing up inside the tissues [estrogen dominance]. Due to the alkaline effect of minerals, they loosen tumors, including fibroid tumors, endometriosis, cysts, moles, warts, skin tags, and other growths, and cause them to release their toxins. The relaxation property of alkaline minerals causes an increase in the bile duct emptying, as is needed with a sluggish gall-bladder. Alkaline substances even loosen fat from cells. In fact, until the body pH reaches 6.4, fat will not budge. Since only alkaline substances [minerals] can neutralize acids, it is clear that minerals are absolutely essential for the health and healing of the body. *pH* [potential of hydrogen concentration] is the term used to identify the intensity of an acid or alkali. The potential ranges from 0 [extremely acidic] to 14 [extremely alkaline]. Optimally, we want the fluids in our bodies to have a neutral pH level, which is 7.0–7.2. No health disorder or disease can possibly sus-tain itself when the pH is maintained in the neutral zone. At this level, the body is highly oxygenated; it detoxifies and heals itself; its cells are ener-gized; and it has a strong immunity to all diseases. A pH less than 5.3 indicates an inability to assimilate vitamins or minerals.

DETOXIFYING TOXIC ELEMENTS WITH CHLORELLA

One of my young patients calls me his "chlorella doctor." I first saw him when he was thirteen and barely functional. His skin was littered with acne. Now sixteen years old, this vaccine-damaged child is able to drive, has an active social life, and is no longer considered mentally challenged. Along with elimi-nating junk foods, adding more fruits and vegetables, a green smoothie, and a probiotic to his diet, I added chlorella. His hair mineral analysis revealed that he was overburdened by toxic mercury, nickel, lead, and antimony. His change each month during metal detoxification was measurable, and he was able to weather the Midwest winters without the constant colds and flu that previ-ously plagued him every year.

Besides binding and removing metals from the body, chlorella research has proven the following benefits: it protects us from radiation; accelerates wound healing, including ulcers; protects us from toxic elements; normalizes digestive and bowel function; retards aging; and stimulates growth and repair of tissues. Research on forty ten-year-old children by Dr. Fujimaki of the people's Sci-entific Research Center in Tokyo demonstrated that the children taking two grams of chlorella daily experienced positive growth and healthy weight gain when compared to a control group. I find that children benefit in many ways—physically, mentally, and emotionally—from taking chlorella daily.

Chlorella is a chelator of heavy metals. The outside shell of Japanese deep-green algae has been fractured so that it is better able to bind and remove toxic metals. Some of the Chinese chlorella does not have a shattered shell and is not as effective a binder for metals. The cell walls of chlorella have three layers: the thick middle layer contains cellulose microfibrils, an outside cell wall, and yet another layer outside the cell wall that contains sporopollenin, a carotenelike active binding substance. Its ability to detoxify chemicals is one of the reasons why chlorella is so powerful. Chlorella is a complete protein: it is 45 percent protein, 20 percent fat, 20 percent carbohydrate, 5 percent fiber, and 10 percent vitamins and minerals. It contains all the B vitamins, plus vitamins C and E, zinc, and iron. Chlorella has an impressive list of health benefits, according to Earl Mindell's *Vitamin Bible*: "It has been found to improve the immune system, improve digestion, detoxify the body and accelerate healing. It can also protect against radiation, aid the prevention of degenerative diseases, help in the treatment of *Candida albicans,* and relieve arthritis pain. Due to its nutritional content, chlorella may also assist in the success of numerous weight loss programs." Chlorella is an effective builder of red blood cells in humans. This provides resistance to infection and promotes good circulation to muscles and the brain.

I suggest the daily use of chlorella for people who might have issues with metals, along with one cup (200 ml) daily of dark green teas, such as nettle or alfalfa. Cilantro is also another raw addition to the diet that stimulates the body to release heavy metals like mercury from the brain and central nervous system into other tissue where it can be bound and removed from the body. As long as we live in a toxic world, I feel that it is essential to add powerful detoxifiers, like chlorella, cilantro, alfalfa, and nettle leaves to our daily diet.

Chlorella is a super protein containing all eight essential amino acids. In the 1970s, a Japanese company devised a way to break down the cell wall of chlorella to make the nutrients more readily available and for it to be easily digested. I have used chlorella since the late eighties to detoxify toxic elements. While dark, raw greens also provide a means of detoxification, chlorella has the added benefit of binding harmful metals in the body and removing them. Research on chlorella has been extensive, although not so much in the United States. In their booklet, "Chlorella," Michael Rosenbaum, M.D., and William H. Lee, R. Ph.D., states: "Until recently, the study of medicinal and nutritional plants was on the decline because pharmaceutical companies—which had worked so energetically to isolate vitamins and other substances from the 1920s to the 1950s—turned their energies into producing synthetic chemicals."

I advise patients to ease into their consumption of chlorella gradually, by taking one of the small tablets for three days and increasing by one every three days until ten are reached. Ten is what I suggest for a 150-pound (68-kg) adult. I would take that amount until a hair mineral analysis demonstrated no toxic elements present in the body. In most cases, it takes over a year if you are an American adult who has consumed a Standard American Diet. I might consider that for every 15 pounds (7 kg) a person might take one chlorella. It can be purchased in tiny tablets, capsules, and powder. I use powdered chlorella in smoothies and take the tablets when we juice. I recommend that patients on a raw diet add this vital nutrient daily to their green smoothie. I would start slowly to minimize the detoxification effects of the powder, beginning with a quarter or half a teaspoon daily and increasing every three days up to two teaspoons (10 ml) daily if it is well-tolerated. Follow the directions on the package for further guidance.

Ten chlorella tablets may contain 1 gram protein, 1,510 IU of vitamin A (as beta-carotene), 2 mg of vitamin C, 38 mcg of B_1, 116 mcg of B_2, 512 mg of niacin (B_3), 48 mcg of B_6, 0.2 mcg of B_{12}, 5 mg of magnesium, 2 mg of iron, 17 mg of potassium, 354 mg of "chlorella growth factor," 76 mg of chlorophyll, and 13 mg of mixed carotenoids. Most chlorella is hypoallergenic and contains no yeast, dairy, egg, gluten, corn, soy, wheat, sugar, starch, salt, preservatives, or artificial color, flavor, or fragrance. It generally contains no binders, dyes, artificial preservatives, carcinogens, or fillers. Check the package to make certain that you are purchasing "broken cell wall" chlorella. Chlorella cannot be consumed raw because, in its natural state, the cell wall has not been altered and it is difficult to digest. Chlorella has five to ten times the amount of chlorophyll as spirulina, but that does not mean that spirulina is not a fantastic adjunct to the raw diet. Spirulina is a multicelled, spiral-shaped plant grown in brackish or salt water. Chlorella is a round, single-celled alga grown in fresh water. For further information about chlorella, I highly recommend Dr. Bernard Jensen's book, *Chlorella: Gem of the Orient.*

CHAPTER 18

Detoxification and Healing Effects

The road to health is the one that begins with an understanding
and commitment to cleanse and detoxify the body,
to restore balance, peace, and harmony.

—BERNARD JENSEN, DC, PH.D.,
THE SCIENCE AND PRACTICE OF IRIDOLOGY, VOL. 1

When I introduce patients to the raw healing diet, I always discuss what they might expect in terms of a healing crisis. Bernard Jensen, DC, Ph.D., once said, "Give me a healing crisis and I can heal any disease." A healing crisis is a good thing. In homeopathy, we always consider the difference between a disease process and a healing crisis. While you may at first associate the feelings or physical, mental, and emotional reactions as the same, they are very different. I relate this healing process as similar to peeling an onion. We strip away old layers of drugs, suppressed diseases, and repressed emotions. If you ever took a drug or an over-the-counter medication, this causes what we call *suppression*. Suppressing a disease only drives it deeper inward and makes you more vulnerable to future disease. It is like layering. And if you throw in drugs and over-the-counter meds, you may find yourself revisiting them and their taste and effects during radical moments of detoxification. Let me give you a quick example. After my first year of raw detoxification, I was stunned by the sudden onset of an excruciating earache. I was overwhelmed by all my feelings of anger and betrayal that my body would dare turn on me when I was so attentive to wellness. As I curled up on the couch with a heating pad on my distressed ear, I had vivid flashbacks to my early childhood when I was

215

plagued with ear infections and tonsillitis. The worst part of this was the help-less feeling and fear I felt. I thought that I was dying, and no one ever told me otherwise. I was retracing—moving back through my disease history—and found myself landing at age three. My great-grandmother had recently died, and I remembered how she curled up on the couch just as I was doing. I could even taste erythromycin antibiotics in my mouth—that is how vivid and nasty the retracing process was. So I am very sensitive to all the symptoms of detoxi-fication that a patient might suffer.

It is useful to learn a bit about natural medicine about Constantine Her-ing's Law of Cure. Constantine Hering was born in Germany on January 1, 1800. He is called the first American homeopath. He researched how people get sick and how they get well. His famous Law of Cure is outlined below.

"We heal from the top to the bottom," Hering said; in other words, from the head down. This has to do with two aspects: the mental and the physical. The mind is a powerful healer. In many ways, it has been concluded that "What the mind can conceive and believe, it can achieve." A positive attitude can create a change in the temperature and healing in a physical being, as has been demonstrated by biofeedback research. In iridology, we notice that Her-ing's Law of Cure does show that healing in the brain itself does occur, espe-cially in its direct relationship with the health of the transverse colon.

"We heal from within to without," Hering noted, or from the inside of us to the outside. This is also known as medial to lateral in anatomical terms. Toxins should be able to leave the body without suppression. In natural medicine, we blame many of our more life-threatening diseases on drug suppression that drives diseases deeper into the body rather than allowing the natural process of elimination to free the body of the toxins. It seems unwise to try to stop the body from doing what it needs to do to heal itself, but that is what over-the-counter medications, aluminum-based commercial deodorants, and most antibiotics do. Mucus, fever, and sweating are the means by which the body gets rid of the root cause of germs, viruses, or toxins that may be present. By suppressing them with drug intervention, these go deeper into the body, causing weaknesses in other areas. A suppressed cold or flu may later settle in the lungs and become bronchitis. Bronchitis suppressed may become pneumonia. Pneu-monia suppressed may become an autoimmune disorder or cancer. Things have to naturally flow out of our body for the body to heal itself.

"We heal in reverse order as the symptoms have appeared," according to Hering's Law of Cure, or the reverse order of the suppression. This means that the last symptom from an infection or disease process will be the first the body deals with as it heals. The body, in its healing, stimulates the immune system to create a fever to burn the toxins out in the following ways:

Through the lungs or bronchioles, causing catarrah or phlegm to be produced.

Through the skin, causing breakouts and rash. This is especially true of detoxification of metals.

Through the colon, eliminating yeast, parasites, old fecal matter, and improperly digested foods.

I have often found that after layers of detoxification, people report disease symptoms that they had when they were seventeen or eighteen. This can be scary to someone who suffered the effects of mononucleosis. If your body reaches the detoxification point of eliminating a deeply suppressed virus, it is wise to acknowledge that you may need to rest. Rest is the first law of healing and the most often ignored. This is unfortunate.

As Constantine Hering theorized, "All healing occurs from the top to the bottom, from the inside out, in the reverse order of the symptoms." From the top down means that all detoxification actually begins with the brain. It is important to be mindful and positive. Affirm that these feelings will pass and detoxification is beneficial and a positive sign that something good is happening through the process. Herxheimer's effect is when toxic materials like yeast die off, cross the brain/blood barrier, and cause a headache or fuzzy thinking. Amazing clarity may follow years of brain fog. While many people tend to think that such brain fog is part of the aging process, it is not. As you detoxify, the mind clears. Rachel, a freshman student in one of my nutrition classes, found it difficult to retain even one sentence of material that she had read. She also struggled to stay awake during class, and I don't think my classes are that boring. Since she had a white-coated tongue, a sign of severe yeast infection, I suggested that she consider a yeast detox and a radical dietary change that included a chef's salad each day, and no dairy, sugar, or bread. Becoming aware of the consequences of a poor diet changed her life. Week after week, she lost pounds and gained more energy. It was not long before she found that her mind was sharper than it had been in nearly a decade. She used her knowledge and enhanced mental capacity to land an upper-management job with a vitamin store chain that she loves.

While fatigue may be symptom of a bad diet, it may also be part of effective dietary detoxification. Many people have a lifetime of suppressed toxins to eliminate, and it does not take much for a minor problem to turn into a major problem. The body is phenomenal at multitasking, but it requires extra energy for healing or fighting the internal effects of eliminating toxins. You may feel exhausted in the process. It is important to listen to what your body needs to recover. Rest is one of the first rules of healing. Unfortunately, it is a rule that many Americans choose to ignore. Pushing your body beyond what it physically can handle in any given day often leads to dire consequences later on. So rest as often as you can during detoxification. There is a point at which energy returns, and you feel an extraordinary surge of it. When my husband and I do a raw juice detox, I have to remind him that when the rush of energy floods in, it must be considered money in the bank that you conserve rather than spend all at once. During this 4-3-2-1 detox, you may also feel a flood of energy. Try not to exhaust it, or yourself. Take it easy until your energy levels balance and reach homeostasis.

If you experience physical pain during detoxification, be aware of where the pain is located and ask yourself what major organs, muscles, or joints may be involved in the aches and pains that you are having. "From the inside out," in Hering's law, indicates that most detoxification or healing begins deep inside and moves outward, from the internal organs outward to the skin. Many people report gastrointestinal or flulike disturbances whenever they change their diet. Such disturbances might include short-term diarrhea or constipation, gas or bloating, or even a feeling of nausea. While you might be intimidated by these, I always feel that your body is just adopting a healing response, rather than **fighting** a disease process. Most of these issues clear within a few days and are actually encouraging of positive change. Why would that be? Because your body finally has a chance to encounter living enzymes, and those enzymes are stirring things up and moving them out. Constipation is a less frequent consequence of detoxification, and a tablespoon (15 ml) of Epsom salt (a natural mineral magnesium sulfate) in eight ounces (227 g) of warm water twice a day will generally assist in getting things moving. I am in favor of weekly colonics or self-administered enemas during the three months you're on this diet. By flushing out the colon, you remove impacted fecal material that prevents the absorption of vitamins and nutrients. You may even be recycling toxins through the bloodstream if you suffer from leaky gut syndrome. Homeopathic remedies are easy to use and understand. I especially like to use them during detoxification because they alleviate symptoms without suppressing detoxification efforts. You can find the best remedy as you check your own symptoms online by visiting abchomeopathy.com. For gut issues, I encourage you to check the remedies Nux vomica or Arsenicum album. It is also useful during this regimen to consume a good probiotic, also known as acidophilus (for the small intestine) and bifidum (for the large intestine.) The small intestine creates probiotics.

You may choose to drink rejeuvelac or take a fructo-oligosaccharide (FOS) free and dairy-free refrigerated probiotic, such as Healthy Trinity by Natren. Also acceptable is a dairy-free probiotic by Garden of Life. We take probiotics (*pro* meaning "for" and *biotic* meaning "life") because in most cases our systems have been gutted of friendly flora by antibiotics. Excessive abuse of antibiotics can cause kidney damage, autoimmune disorders like fibromyalgia and multiple sclerosis, and leaky gut. Joint and muscle pain is fairly common during detoxification, for the joints and muscles are forced to give up some of their xenotoxins during the enzyme-flooding stage. Extra essential fatty acids in the diet nurture the joints. Soaking in a warm bathtub with two cups of Epsom salts will help sore muscles and joints relax and release stress.

Emotional distress, including irritability and mood swings, may also be a part of the detoxification process. Again, I might refer you to homeopathic remedies that might make it easier for you to tolerate your symptoms. If you know your homeopathic constitution, taking your remedy would be the best approach. Part of the negative emotions that you experience may be related to cravings coming from the monster xenobiotics inside you, demanding to be fed. These critters thrive on sugar, fructose, gluten, and yeast.

I find it useful to encourage individuals who are changing their diet or detoxifying to discuss the possibility of irritability with their families. Ask them not to take personally any excessive anger or crying that you may experience during this process. Warn them that you may not be quite your normal, casual, balanced self, but that you might need extra support and understanding in the next three months. Ask them not to sabotage your efforts. It is a sad fact that misery loves company, and as you get more energetic and healthy, some people in your social circle might be a bit jealous and critical of your healing efforts. They might even bring you a box of your favorite doughnuts. Remember to share some dietary guidelines or boundaries with friends and relatives before you begin. If you are attending a social function, it is not a bad idea to take your own food or snacks along. There are great soft-sided mini totes that can keep your delicious veggie treats cool. Two sisters on the raw diet discovered that they always had to take extra raw treats along for all those curious friends who wanted to try whatever snacks or meals they had prepared! They now have a raw catering business in Chicago.

Keeping a positive attitude and allowing your emotions to surface affirms that you are choosing to nurture and understand more of what you are feeling and experiencing. Stuffing emotions is as toxic as stuffing doughnuts. They often lead to the same weight issue. One of the affirmations I like is this: "I love myself enough to eat raw organic foods. I take time to select and enjoy delicious, enzyme-rich foods. I deserve to feel good and be healthy. I nurture myself with raw organic fruits and vibrant vegetables, nuts, seeds, and grains. I care for myself. I am tuned in to my emotions and know how good I feel when I eat what feeds my body, mind, spirit, and emotions. I release my addiction to toxic foods. I recognize and avoid foods that harm me. I am a good steward of my body. I have fun with delicious healthy foods." Affirmations work when you repeat them frequently and embrace their truth. Please feel free to formulate your own positive words to feed your emotional needs. In the past, you may have viewed any change in old dietary habits as punishment. It is time to understand that what you were doing was following a mindless pattern created by careless, greedy industries. Do not be a pawn to their greed. Put your adult self in charge of making sound decisions. The child in you may throw a tantrum for sugar, but if you love yourself enough, you will make good healing decisions for a change. One of the affirmations for the adult in you might be: "In the past I made poor food choices to feed the emotional needs in me that were not being fed. I now recognize that what I hunger most for is love. Food is not a substitute for love. Now I eat good food as fuel for health. I love and accept myself and I nurture my inner child with wisdom and vibrant food choices. I feed my inner child love and enzyme-rich food that will make us both feel better. I release any hidden desire to punish myself from my past. I put the adult self in charge, and I know what is healthy, whole, and nurturing. I love myself and nurture myself with adult food choices. I put the adult me in charge of selecting and eating good food. I keep in my house only nurturing, healthy foods."

White tongue and extra mucus or catarrh can also signal extreme and beneficial detoxification. I remember learning decades ago from classes with the famous German healer Hannah Kroeger that the disease of cancer begins with excessive yeast overgrowth in the body. Medical research in other countries is now revealing that this is an underlying cause. In Oriental medicine, the etiology of fibromyalgia is considered yeast overgrowth. You may scrape the tongue with a tongue scraper designed for that purpose, or use the concave edge of a tablespoon or teaspoon to scrape as far back on the tongue as you can and then rinse the tongue. Use natural tooth oil to avoid demineralization of the tooth enamel. I also suggest the Ayurvedic principle of oil pulling prior to brushing the teeth or eating anything, first thing in the morning after rising from bed.

OIL PULLING ORAL DETOX

Upon rising: Take one teaspoon (5 ml) of raw coconut or sesame oil and swish it for five to ten minutes. Spit the bacteria-laden oil in the toilet bowl. Rinse with one teaspoon (5 ml) of baking soda dissolved in half a cup (100 ml) of warm water. Brush teeth and tongue.

One woman's husband thanked me for sharing this oral detox recipe with his wife. He declared that he had ten minutes of peace in the morning. The couple had a delightful relationship. The thrush-coated tongue is a good sign; detoxifying internal body cavities ensures that you are sloughing off disease-causing antigens, bacteria, and old, dead cellular material. Yeast die-off occurs naturally during the 4-3-2-1 raw diet. Excessive mucus released through a runny nose or during fecal eliminations is simply your body's way of expelling toxins. A headache is often common during this time. Again, this should pass within a few days. Drinking more water or a warm cup of Pau D'Arco tea helps to move toxins out of the body and keeps you feeling full and your joints hydrated. Warm ginger packs on the stomach and abdominal area reduce cool dampness and colon discomfort. You may make a cup (200 ml) of raw ginger tea: one tablespoon (15 ml) of raw grated ginger in one cup (200 ml) of boiling water. Steep for five minutes and then strain away the ginger pulp. Soak a washcloth in the tea and place it flat on the stomach area, centering it directly on the naval. Put a hot water bottle or warm heating pad on top of the wash-cloth and rest for fifteen minutes. Another method is to place six drops of gin-ger essential oil around your naval and massage this in with deep circles. If you are sensitive or have environmental allergies, I suggest massaging in castor oil or olive oil on the naval area first. Place a warm, damp washcloth on the area and then a warm heating pad or hot water bottle. Again, I recommend that you rest for fifteen minutes. Ginger in any form is contraindicated if you have high blood pressure. You may also ask your health care professional to adjust your ileocecal valve and teach you how to maintain its integrity or adjust it yourself. There are also techniques for this that are shared previously. You might google the words *ileocecal valve* or *IC valve adjustment* for photos if you need them.

While detoxification is not generally a pleasant experience, I would ask that you consider the alternative. We clean and disinfect the inside of our houses, our cars, and even our refrigerators. You are probably long overdue for an internal cleansing of your body. Medical treatments or pharmaceutical drugs for most life-threatening diseases can take a lifetime, may compromise your immune system, harm vital organs, cause hair loss, shorten your life expectancy, force you to draw blood and take injections several times a day, and leave you feeling much worse than the few days of detoxification that you might expect. Give this simple three-month program a try and see how it reverses aging and restores health. Most important of all, don't give up because you are detoxifying.

NATURAL DEODORANT RECIPES

COCONUT BASE

Ingredients

¼ cup (50 ml) aluminum-free baking soda

¼ cup (50 ml) arrowroot powder *or* corn starch (mix with above)

5 tablespoons (75 ml) pure organic coconut oil

Variation: Add 2 tablespoons (30 ml) extra-virgin olive oil

Directions

Blend coconut oil (and olive oil, if you're using it) slowly into the dry ingredients, making a paste. Press into a container. Apply with clean hands or a tongue depressor.

DRY BASE DEODORANT

This is the recipe I teach students during lymphatic classes to help prevent cancer.

Ingredients

1 cup (200 ml) aluminum-free baking soda

Directions

Dust on powder with a cotton ball or shake it into your clean hands and apply. If a rash develops due to detoxification of yeast, stop it at once, take probiotics orally, and apply some probiotics to the underarms with water or coconut oil. Avoid overwashing and allow a few days of bare underarms for this to heal. It is best if you shave your underarms to allow eight hours before applying any type of deodorant application. Thai stones may contain aluminum and might trigger this type of detoxification as well.

IF A HEALING CRISIS OCCURS	
Loose stools	Fairly common early in detox; eat $1/2$ banana, drink more water; dissolve 2 tablespoons (30 ml) Bentonite clay in water.
Sinus or mucus	Catarrah is part of detox of the colon; let it flow. Elevate your head at night.
Headache	Sinus congestion or constipation. Dissolve 1 teaspoon (5 ml) Epsom salts in 10 ounces water; drink 1 cup (200 ml) Pau D'Arco tea.
Hypoglycemia	Eat a few soaked nuts with fruit. Eat more frequently—every 2 hours or so.
Energy drops in the evening	Blood sugar drops (see Hypoglycemia above)
Constipation	Sluggish transverse colon. Hydrocolon therapy or enema. Consume senna tea or Epsom salts in water.
Feeling grouchy	Cellular and emotional detox. Yoga, walking, exercise. Eat more vitamin B–rich vegetables or cacao.
Anger	Counseling, inner child work. Take a 4,000 mg B_{12} supplement.
Can't sleep	Signals an immune response and/or inflammation. Chamomile tea, 5HTP, more morning exercise, melatonin or tryptophan, and an apple in the evening.
Excessive weight loss	Common in the first 2 months. Patience: Weight will stabilize.
Weight plateaus	Common during program. Patience: Weight will stabilize.

It is a sad and sorry fact that the average weight of Americans is increasing. According to the National Center for Health Statistics, the average weight for an adult female in the United States in 2008 was 162.9 pounds (74 kg), average height 5-foot-4. The average for men 5-foot-9 is 190 pounds (86 kg). The National Health and Nutrition Examination Survey 2001–2004 states that:

The average weight for men aged 20–74 years rose dramatically from 166.3 pounds in 1960 to 191 pounds in 2002, while the average weight for women the same age increased from 140.2 pounds in 1960 to 164.3 pounds in 2002.

The average weight for a 10-year-old-boy in 1963 was 74.2 pounds; by 2002, the average weight was nearly 85 pounds.

The average weight for a 10-year-old girl in 1963 was 77.4 pounds; by 2002, the average weight was nearly 88 pounds.

A 15-year-old boy weighed 135.5 pounds on average in 1966; by 2002, the average weight of a boy that age increased to 150.3 pounds.

A 15-year-old girl weighed 124.2 pounds on average in 1966; by 2002, the average weight for a girl that age was 134.4 pounds. While about two-thirds of adults in the United States are overweight, a frightening one-third are obese.

This fact sheet, available online, presents statistics on overweight and obesity in the United States, as well as health risks, mortality rates, and economic costs associated with these conditions. In the January 28, 2009, *Health Day News,* it was reported that almost 13 percent of adults twenty and older have diabetes, and another 40 percent have not yet been diagnosed. This is related to excessive weight and bad diet as well as a lack of exercise. According to the National Eating and Disorders Association, Americans spend more than $40 billion a year on dieting and diet-related products, while avoiding expert opinions to increase exercise to thirty minutes five days per week. The association states that "carrying extra pounds leads to an increased risk of heart disease, diabetes, stroke, arthritis, depression, and cancer."

I consider diabetes to be a life-threatening disease that leads to kidney and heart failure. It can most often be reversed with a raw diet and exercise. It is now considered to be unhealthy to be thin or even at your optimum weight.

When you are on a raw diet for more than two months, it is common for fat to drop from your body. One of my patients' coworkers were extremely upset that she was shedding pounds when they could not. She was reported to human resources because they feared that she had a major disease. She was forced to take two weeks off without pay to "rehabilitate." Even though she explained that she was on a healing diet and had never in her life felt better, she was shunned because she was achieving what her coworkers could not—optimum health. She was a mere five feet tall and had lost thirty pounds (13.5 kg). She still weighed 130 pounds (59 kg).

LIVER DETOXIFICATION

Sick foods that are poor quality or too rich and fatty stress the liver. This pressure on the liver leads to a decreased ability to manufacture bile and clear excess toxins and hormones. Antioxidant-rich foods like raw fruits and vegetables protect the liver and keep it healthy and they act as binders to cleanse and detoxify the liver.

Foods That Protect and Detoxify the Liver

Beets, carrots, eggplant, and red onions contain flavonoids and beta-carotene, which are powerful antioxidants that help detoxify the liver. Grapefruit is also high in antioxidants.

Apple pectin (apples) binds and helps excrete heavy metals directly from the intestines. This reduces the filtration load on the liver.

Garlic and its allicin with the mineral selenium remove heavy metals from the liver.

Spinach and broccoli contain B-complex vitamins that improve liver function and promote liver decongestion.

Other cruciferous vegetables, including cauliflower, cabbage, and broccoli, contain glucosinolates that help the liver produce enzymes for detoxification.

Dandelion, artichoke, and mustard greens promote bile production and flow.

CHAPTER 19

Raw Eliminations

How do you know that enzymes are working? What you will experience is an increase in formed bowel movements—at least 1 to 2 times a day, usually after every meal—"one meal in, one meal out." Also, these movements will not have a foul odor. When this happens, it means your food is being digested properly and used by your body instead of sitting in your intestines to rot and putrefy.

—EDWARD HOWELL, *ENZYME NUTRITION*

I would like you give you the following useful information about your eliminations. A healthy bowel movement should not take much time to release and remove from your sigmoid colon. In an ideal world, mammals should have a bowel movement right after they eat a regular meal. If you find that you do not have at least one bowel movement per day, you are probably constipated or have a delayed transit time. A prolapsed transverse colon is a situation where the colon droops because it has had the burden of too much weight for too long a time. A prolapsed transverse colon always puts pressure on the organs that lie beneath it, and this can stimulate unhealthy disease processes in those organs. Another unfortunate event that occurs with a congested colon or congestion in the hepatic or splenic flexures, the curve in the upper right and left part of the transverse colon, is that you can create an environment for opportunistic bad yeasts like *Candida albicans* or parasites to reside. A disease process called "cool dampness" may follow. I always tell patients to imagine what it would be like to drive a car where you never clean the inside or eliminate the trash that you accumulate. If you have that car for a few years, it gets full of trash, especially if you regularly eat in your car or at drive-through food restaurants. We have to take out the trash in our colon, and eating raw foods helps to ensure that enough fiber is consumed on a regular basis to clear out digestive problems. In fact, one of the major changes that most people rave about to me is their new and improved bowel habits. One man said to me: "I used to make myself go once a week, and it was a strain and a struggle to get out a few marble-sized nuggets. Now I am in and out before I can even read the first page of the paper. I don't bother taking the paper into the bathroom with me anymore."

Listed below are the types of stool as is measured by what is called the Bristol Stool Scale. There are charts available online for you if you are curious about pictures that illustrate the seven types of stool. It was developed as a measure of health or disease based on the shape and consistency of fecal matter. We must get curious about our eliminations if we are going to be serious about our health. I tell patients, just glance down before you flush. It is more than interesting the stories that I get back about what people leave behind. I feel that lumpy, hard stools are part of a sluggish transverse colon. If things do not improve drastically after a month of raw foods, I would encourage anyone to consider colon hydrotherapy, also called colonics, or the use of a colema board for enemas weekly that can be purchased online. Until we begin to understand that health involves encouraging the intake of more enzymes and at least one good, productive, S-shaped bowel movement, one to two inches (2.5–5 cm) around, per day, adults are at risk for disease processes.

The Bristol Stool Scale, or the Bristol Stool Chart, is a medical aid designed to classify the form of human feces into seven categories. It is sometimes referred to in the United Kingdom as the Meyers Scale. It was developed by Dr. Ken Heaton and S. J. Lewis at the University of Bristol, and was first published in the *Scandinavian Journal of Gastroenterology* in 1997. The form of the stool depends on the time it spends in the colon.

The Seven Types of Stool in the Bristol Scale

Type 1: Separate hard lumps, like nuts (hard to pass)

Type 2: Sausage-shaped, but lumpy

Type 3: Like a sausage but with cracks on its surface (ideal)

Type 4: Like a sausage or snake, smooth and soft (ideal)

Type 5: Soft blobs with clear-cut edges (passed easily)

Type 6: Fluffy pieces with ragged edges, a mushy stool

Type 7: Entirely liquid

Types 1 and 2 indicate constipation. Types 3 and 4 represent the "ideal stools" especially the latter, as they are the easiest to pass from the body. Types 5 to 7 are tending toward diarrhea or urgency that means a disease or parasite may be a problem.

BENTONITE CLAY

Bentonite clay is found in Utah, formed from a layer of volcanic ash that fell into a shallow inland sea. As this ash filtered through seawater, it formed a layer of pure minerals that dried into clay. While Bentonite is not considered part of the traditional raw diet, I consider it highly beneficial for its ability to remove toxins and parasites from the colon and expedite healing processes. It also helps provide easily absorbed ferrous and ferric iron to help cure anemia. By neutralizing allergens, it reduces allergic reactions; it also reduces heartburn and indigestion by absorbing excess stomach acids. As it goes through the colon, the clay scrapes and cleans the lining of the small and large intestines, increasing its ability to absorb minerals and other nutrients, and making the minerals even more bioavailable for absorption. One type of Bentonite contains seventy-one trace as well as ultratrace minerals, such as ruthenium, tellurium, and thulium. Trace minerals enable the body to absorb nutrients as they act as bonding agents between you and your food. Research published in *Medical Annals of the District of Columbia* in 1961 by Frederic Damrau, M.D., established the ability of Bentonite clay to end diarrhea. Thirty-five people with diarrhea took two tablespoons (30 ml) of Bentonite in distilled water daily. Ninety-seven percent of the patients were relieved of symptoms in 3.8 days. Regardless of the problem—allergies, spastic colon, viral infection, or food poisoning—the use of Bentonite proved highly effective and safe.

For detoxification and diarrhea relief, the best way to ingest Bentonite is on an empty stomach an hour before or after eating. I prefer to launch into Bentonite clay with 1 tablespoon (15 ml) daily mixed in water or a bit of raw apple juice. Try this for one week and then increase by one tablespoon (15 ml) each week (up to a maximum of four divided doses daily) to your tolerance. Twice a year, I would consider a four-week Bentonite cleanse. It is also available in capsules.

BENTONITE MUD PACK
FOR EXTERNAL DETOXIFYING

Bentonite clay may be made into a paste to place on the abdomen or stomach to relieve inflammatory processes. The paste is made by mixing a few drops of ginger or basil oil and water, together with the clay and some powdered herbs or a few drops of basil or ginger essential oil. Make a mud pack and rub it onto your stomach and abdomen. Apply heat for about ten minutes. Put on an old tank top or shirt and go to bed. In the morning shower it off.

DR. MITCHELL'S COLON CLEANSE POWDER

Ingredients

2 cups psyllium husk whole

$\frac{1}{2}$ cup Bentonite clay

$\frac{1}{8}$ cup senna

Additions: I generally use two or three of the following extras in powder form to the above recipe according to each individual:

2 T each: chlorella (to detoxify metals), magnesium citrate (to retain more water in the small intestine), L-glutamine (to assist inflammation in the small intestine), slippery elm (for irritable bowel), fennel (for gas), haritaki (for bacteria), triphala (for added bowel stimulation), bromelain (for inflammation)

Directions: Add 1 teaspoon of the colon cleanse powder to your smoothie, or stir in warm water or water plus two packages of Emergen-C Lite with MSM. After two weeks, try to take one teaspoon in the morning and one in the afternoon.

CHAPTER 20

Beverages

Drinking a daily cup of tea will surely starve the apothecary.
—CHINESE PROVERB

I mentioned that nettle and alfalfa tea is useful in the detoxification of xeno-toxic metals from the body. Alfalfa is also good for individuals who have high cholesterol. Nettle is high in iron for people who are anemic or iron-deficient.

Green tea is high in polyphenols, and it has antioxidant properties. The FDA has concluded that green tea drinkers may be reducing their risk for breast and prostate cancer. Research done by Yale University hypothesized that "1.2 liters of green tea consumed daily might provide high levels of polyphenols and other antioxidants that improve cardiovascular health and counteract the negative effects of smoking." Other studies indicate that because tea is high in anti-inflammatory properties, tea extracts might be effective in treating patients who suffer from damaged skin following radiation treatments for cancer. Drinking green tea to excess may cause liver toxicity and oxidative stress, and some medical doctors claim that pregnant women should avoid green tea altogether.

Pau D'Arco tea is one that I often suggest for patients who are on a yeast detoxification diet or if they are plagued by gastrointestinal issues. I have found it particularly useful to mitigate the Herxheimer's reaction, including headache and brain detoxification. Recent studies have been conducted on the lapachol molecule found in tabebuia as an anticancer agent. It has been used around the world for various herbal treatments, and in Brazilian herbal medicine (the bark is grown in Brazil) it is considered an astringent, antifungal, anti-inflammatory, and antibacterial beverage. It has been used to treat ulcers, boils, dysentery, leukemia, diabetes, syphilis, urinary tract infections, gastro-intestinal and yeast issues, cancer, allergies, and constipation.

If you have backaches, I encourage you to consider drinking one cup (200 ml) daily of kidney tea blend. This is one tablespoon (15 ml) of the mix of equal parts of dried roots of hydrangea, marshmallow, and gravel root. Pour hot water into a quart jar over the herbs and allow the mixture to steep over night. Drain, and refrigerate the root mixture. Drink the tea slowly or it might cause gastric upset.

A great herbal tea for intestinal distress and gas is also considered a spice for the kitchen: fennel. You simply add one teaspoon (5 ml) of ground fennel seeds to a cup (200 ml) of hot water, steep, and strain. Drink once or twice a day. Chronic flatulence is often attributed to bowel pockets. A raw diet and colon detoxification measures enable these pockets to heal. Sometimes hip pain may accompany bowel pockets. Eliminating those can free you of those aches.

Bitters tea is one of my favorites for patients with stomach or gastric issues. Drinking half a cup (100 ml) prior to meals is best, or during or after meals if that is all that works for you. It contains any combination or these simple herbs: gentian root, dandelion root, cardamom, fennel, angelica, and orange peel (go lightly on this). Combine equal parts of all but the orange peel; that would be one-fourth of the quantity of any of the others.

Parasite teas generally contain herbs called vermifuges. My recipe for Quad Para tea is as follows:

$1/2$ cup each of black walnut leaf, quassia bark, and Pau D'Arco bark. $1/8$ cup of Wormwood, and 2 T chopped pumpkin seeds. Mix all and add 2 T of the blend to a quart of very hot water. Allow to steep overnight, then strain. Once a day, drink one cup slowly for eighteen days. Refrigerate. I also make a tincture of the above if tea is undesirable. For tapeworms, a twenty-four-hour fast, drinking only four ounces of cucumber juice plus four ounces of water with four tablespoons of raw honey, may be benefi-cial. Follow with three cups of senna-pumpkin seed tea made with one teaspoon of senna and 2 tablespoons of crushed or chopped pumpkin seeds. Steep tea for fifteen minutes, strain and then drink. Expect strong evacuation and evidence of tapeworms expelled. Tapeworms in the liver have been mistaken in the past for cancer.

CHAPTER 21

Getting Ready to Go Raw

Before everything else, getting ready is the secret to success.

—HENRY FORD

As you prepare to begin the 4-3-2-1 healing diet, I would like to encourage you to educate yourself more about the long-term health benefits of a raw healing diet. Select one of the many available raw preparation books on the market today to create delicious and nutritious meals. Recipes may feature options that I have not mentioned, including the use of oils, spices, and even natural sources of sugar. Just because I do not place them into one of the categories does not mean that you must exclude them from your culinary creations. In fact, in the colder climates I encourage the use of spices like ginger and chilies to warm digestion in the winter months.

Oils are important, but please vary your use of them. Remember to employ olive, flax, and sesame oils. If you use sweeteners, like dates, honey, maple syrup, molasses, and agave nectar, please use them sparingly and not on a daily basis in the three months of this healing diet. Sweeteners must be pure, with no sugar additives.

Make this healing lifestyle an adventure. Allow yourself to have fun with this new information about what food is and does. Really learn what food does in and to your body and how it creates your future life. All your activities and emotions in life are fueled by the food you eat. This is just the beginning of your new quality of life.

When I first switched to a raw foods diet, I was motivated and excited to try new recipes. I was not a gourmet cook, but I embraced the fun and ease of raw food preparation. I enjoyed trying new raw food recipes from books or online resources. I learned that raw food preparation is not rocket science. I was relieved that I could make tasty and healthy creations from simple, fresh produce and fruit. It is empowering to try something new in your life. If you have been intimidated in the past by change, just tell yourself that you are open to this new beginning, this healing chapter in your life. If I can do this, you can, too. You can choose very easy, quick recipes from *Alive in Five,* or more difficult ones to please your inner gourmet chef. Cleanup is easy because there are no greasy, burned pans to scrub. One woman in our raw potluck group even donated her kitchen stove to Habitat for Humanity because she never intended to use it again. That was several years ago, and she now has enough space to dine in her small kitchen and look out the window. She delights in how one person can create delicious meals for one with no waste and very little time.

I will share a few of my own personal quick recipes and a simple sample shopping list for one week that I often use. I owe the foundation of these creative ideas to brave, raw pioneers who first researched this path. It is time for you to develop your own variations to the field of greens.

CHAPTER 22

A–Z Master Organic Grocery List

I've been making a list of the things they don't teach you at school.

—NEIL GAIMAN

Choose the amount of leafy greens, cruciferous vegetables, seeds, or nuts for one week and buy only what you need. No preprepared produce products.

Note: Nothing on this list is to be cooked, and all should be organic.

Print or copy this list and circle only the items you need each week before shopping.

AMOUNT	FOOD
6	Apples: Granny Smith, Fuji, Braeburn, Cortland
2 cups (400 ml)	Almonds, raw, nonirradiated are best
1 jar	Almond or cashew butter, one of either; make sure the label says *raw*
1 quart (1 liter)	Apple cider vinegar as a fruit and vegetable wash—2 tablespoons (30 ml) to 1 gallon (4 liters) of water
7–8	Avocados—some black and ready to eat; some more green to ripen
1 bunch	Basil, fresh or in a container to add to salads or use in paté recipe
1	Beet to use in salad or in smoothies or to juice
1–2	Blueberries: fresh or organic frozen containers or bags

AMOUNT	FOOD
1 bottle	Bragg Aminos or Nama Shoyu, for seasoning
1 small package	Brazil nuts for selenium
1 head	Broccoli
12	Carrots, medium to large, not in package is best
1 bag	Cashews, raw in bag (cashews are never really raw, use not roasted)
1 small head	Cauliflower
1 head	Purple or green cabbage or kale or collard greens
1 bunch	Cilantro to make guacamole or use in smoothies or salads
1 bunch	Celery, not in package is best; use for smoothies or stuff with almond or cashew butter
2 ears	Corn on the cob or 1 package frozen organic corn; use for salad
1 jar	Cumin: dry, ground cumin for seasoning
1 package	Edamame, frozen or fresh as quick snack (fresh must be flash-boiled)
1 bulb	Fennel; fresh for salads
1 package	Flax seeds, ground in spice grinder and added to salads, smoothies, or recipes
2	Grapefruit; pink is best to eat fresh or use in salads
4 bulbs	Garlic to use in recipes
1 small bunch	Grapes, purple seedless, to eat as snacks
1	Ginger root to use in recipes, smoothies, and grated 1 tablespoon (15 ml) to make a cup of tea
1 box or bag	Green tea
1 carton or bunch	Green beans, to eat as snack raw or to use in salads
1 bag	Hemp seeds
1 jar	Italian seasoning spice to use in recipes or salad dressing
1	Jicama, small, to slice for snacks or use on salads
1 bunch	Kale or collards greens, cabbage, or napa (rotate each week to diversify)

Amount	Food
2	Lemons and/or limes to use in recipes
1 bag	Dried lentils to sprout to use in recipes
1	Mango, dried or whole, to eat as a snack or to add to recipes
1	Mesculin salad or other fresh salad greens as spinach or field greens
1	Napa cabbage or some other cabbage to use in recipes for crunch
1 package	Nori to add to green smoothie or as a wrap for raw vegan sushi
2	Oranges to use as snack or in recipes (use only if your body is yeast-free)
1	Papaya; use fruit and cut up for next week; use seeds for salad dressing
4	Peaches
2	Pears for smoothie (use pear with apple if you're constipated), as fruit snack
1 package	Pecans to use in recipes or as snack; may substitute for any nuts
1	Pau D'Arco tea to drink as beverage, a bark tea with mild flavor
1	Pineapple, small, or 1 small container to use as snack for fruit for 2 weeks
1 small package	Pine nuts to use in recipes or on salads
1 small package	Pumpkin seeds 1 package
	Quinoa to sprout (sprouts overnight and can be eaten the next day)
1	Red leaf lettuce, to be eaten as salad or used in smoothies
4	Romaine lettuce heads to use in smoothies or salads or as a wrap for paté
1	Small bag of seaweed or sea vegetables; bag or shaker if used as salt
1 head	Spinach or container of baby leaf, for use as salad or in smoothies
1 jar	Tahini to use in recipes or smoothies
2	Zucchini or summer squash to use in recipes or as a raw pasta

SHORT ORGANIC SHOPPING LIST FOR SMOOTHIES OR JUICING	
AMOUNT	**FOOD**
2 heads	Leafy green lettuce (red leaf, green leaf, romaine); no iceberg
1 bunch	Spinach (if your kidneys are not an issue for you)
1 bunch	Carrots, approximately 12–18
3	Cucumbers
1 bunch	Celery
1 bunch	Cilantro or parsley (really good for kidneys)
1 bunch	Red radishes (about 6) if your thyroid is an issue
2	Each of pear and/or Granny Smith apples
1	Raw ginger root (if high blood pressure is not an issue); you may also use this for tea
1 jar	Cinnamon (not cassia)

CHAPTER 23

Simple Recipe Suggestions: Monday Through Sunday

*Maybe a person's time would be as well spent
raising food as raising money to buy food.*

—FRANK A. CLARK

EASY 4-3-2-1 RAW FASTING RECIPES FOR ONE PERSON

Breakfast Monday

AVOCADO SMASH

Directions

Smash with fork: 1 avocado and $1/2$ banana. Top with $1/3$ cup (68 ml) berries

Optional: Add 1 tablespoon (15 ml) ground hemp or flax and/or 1 teaspoon (5 ml) of organic cinnamon.

Lunch Monday

SALAD

Directions

2–3 cups of leafy greens of choice with fresh dill or basil, chopped broccoli, carrots, olive oil, sunflower, and lemon juice salad dressing (see Simple Salad Dressing on page 246).

Optional: You may add Nama Shoyu to the dressing.

Dinner Monday

SERIOUS GARDEN MELANGE

Ingredients

6 asparagus spears cut into 1-inch (2.5-cm) pieces

$1/2$–1 zucchini or summer squash diced thick

$1/2$ cup (100 ml) chopped tomato

1 cup (200 ml) chopped endive or collard greens

5 chopped kalamata olives

$1/2$ cup (100 ml) macadamia or cashew nuts.

Directions

Mix all ingredients and top with dressing.

Set to soak: 1 cup (200 ml) lentils, 2 cups (400 ml) sunflower seeds, 1 cup (200 ml) alfalfa seeds, 1 cup (200 ml) rinsed quinoa, and 4 tablespoons (60 ml) (or more if you'd like some for snacks) nuts for breakfast fruit on Tuesday.

Breakfast Tuesday

Directions

Take 2 cups (400 ml) of chopped fruit in season and top with 4 tablespoons (60 ml) nuts soaked overnight and 1 tablespoon (15 ml) cinnamon.

Lunch Tuesday

QUINOA SALAD

Directions

Rinse and drain sprouted quinoa seeds. Add $1/2$ cup (50 ml) chopped cilantro, $1/2$ chopped avocado, 1 cup (200 ml) shelled edamame or fresh or frozen peas. You may add spices of your choice, including chili. Dress with Simple Salad Dressing (see page 246).

Dinner Tuesday

LENTIL TACOS

Ingredients

1 cup (200 ml) sprouted lentils or raw corn

1 clove garlic, pressed

8 chopped black sun-dried olives

½ avocado or ½ tomato, cubed

¼ cup (50 ml) fresh chopped cilantro

2 teaspoons (10 ml) curry powder or Italian herbs

1 tablespoon (15 ml) olive oil

3 whole romaine leaves

Directions

Stir all ingredients together and stuff romaine leaves with the mixture.

Breakfast Wednesday

BLENDER GREEN DRINK

(FOR MORE IDEAS SEE *GREEN FOR LIFE* BY VICTORIA BOUTENKO.)

Directions

Blend ½ avocado, 4–6 leaves of romaine lettuce or 1 cup (200 ml) spinach leaves, 2 kale or collard green leaves, 1–2 cups (200–400 ml) cold water, 1 tablespoon (15 ml) cinnamon, 1 teaspoon (5 ml) grated raw ginger, 1 sheet of nori or 1 tablespoon (15 ml) dulse or kelp.

Lunch Wednesday

STUFFED TOMATO

Directions

Core and cut in half 1 large tomato (you could use red pepper in this recipe) and stuff with Sunflower Paté (see recipe on following page).

SUNFLOWER PATÉ

Ingredients

2 cups sunflower seeds, soaked overnight and rinsed

$1/2$ cup (100 ml) lemon juice

$1/4$ cup (50 ml) nut butter, like almond or tahini

3 tablespoons (45 ml) cilantro or parsley

1 teaspoon (5 ml) Nama Shoya (optional)

Directions

Blend all ingredients in a food processor until you like the texture. You may refrigerate any leftovers for dinner on Sunday.

Dinner Wednesday

LAYERED SALAD

Directions

In a food processor with an S-blade, lightly pulse the following starchy vegetables: $1/2$ cup (100 ml) broccoli, $1/2$ cup (100 ml) cauliflower, 4 leaves each of kale or collards, 3 celery stalks, $1/2$ red bell pepper. You may add some minced onion, garlic, or ginger, if you'd like. Top with cashew dressing or any other dressing of your choice.

Breakfast Thursday

DR. MITCHELL'S ORGANIC BLENDER SMOOTHIE

Blend the following:

Ingredients

1 Granny Smith or Fuji apple or 1 pear
(if you're constipated)

2 stalks of celery

$1/2$ avocado

Leafy greens, including 2–3 leaves of romaine lettuce or 2 cups (400 ml)
any leafy greens and sprouts (You may also use or include cruciferous
greens like collard greens or kale—no mustard greens.)

$\frac{1}{2}$ tablespoon (8 ml) raw ginger, peeled (You can grate or use
pieces that are peeled. This can be a $\frac{1}{4}$-inch [6 mm] thick piece.
Avoid ginger if you have high blood pressure.)

1 cup (200 ml) purified water

1 large carrot (avoid carrots if you have cancer)

1 tablespoon (15 ml) cinnamon and or agave nectar

Directions

Blend all ingredients until smooth.

Additions to the above smoothie recipe may include 1 tablespoon (15 ml)
each dulse or kelp (or 1 sheet of raw nori,) ground raw flax, ground
sesame seeds, Japanese chlorella, L-glutamine, magnesium citrate powder,
or colon cleanse powder.

Lunch Thursday

HUMMUS DIPPERS

Cut slices of starchy vegetables, like carrots, red bell pepper, celery stalks,
and cucumber strips. Dip in hummus.

Ingredients

1 cup (200 ml) frozen (thawed)
or sprouted chickpeas or sprouted lentils

$\frac{1}{4}$ cup (50 ml) sesame tahini

2 tablespoons (30 ml) Simple Salad Dressing

$\frac{1}{4}$ teaspoon (1 ml) cumin powder

1 clove garlic

$\frac{1}{4}$ cup (50 ml) parsley or cilantro

Sea salt to taste, or 1 teaspoon (5 ml) Bragg Aminos

Directions

Blend until smooth.

Dinner Thursday

LIGHT AND CRUNCHY SALAD

Ingredients

2 cups mixed green salad, dressed

$1/2$ julienned zucchini or summer squash and bell pepper

$1/2$ cup (100 ml) chopped broccoli or any other starchy vegetables of your choice

Directions

Marinate in almond butter dressing: take 1 tablespoon (15 ml) sesame oil, 1 teaspoon (5 ml) Bragg Aminos, and 3 tablespoons (45 ml) almond butter; add Thai curry or any warm spices. Top with nuts, hemp seeds, or ground flax.

Breakfast Friday

APPLE BOATS

Directions

Cut in half and remove seeds from 1 apple. Fill it with raw almond or cashew butter. Top with raisins.

Lunch Friday

MISO OR SEAWEED SOUP

Directions

Mix salad greens (2 cups [400 ml]) with $1/2$ cup (50 ml) alfalfa sprouts and 1 cup (200 ml) starchy vegetable chunks, like jicama. Add finely chopped garlic, broccoli, or kale. Top with pine nuts or sea vegetables. Add dressing of your choice.

Dinner Friday

SLICED PORTOBELLO STEAK

Directions

Remove stem. Clean thoroughly outside and underside (removing gills) of portabella with a paper towel soaked in vinegar water. Slice into thin strips and marinate for 15 minutes in 6 tablespoons (90 ml) Simple Salad Dressing, adding spices of your choice, such as garlic. Layer onto 2 cups (400 ml) of mixed greens, tossed with dressing.

Breakfast Saturday

FROZEN FRUIT SMOOTHIE

Directions

Blend $1/2$ frozen banana, 1 cup (200 ml) frozen fruit organic, $1/2$ cup (100 ml) cold almond milk, young coconut milk, or sesame milk.

Breakfast Sunday

DR. MITCHELL'S SESAME, BANANA, BLUEBERRY SHAKE TO WAKE UP

Directions

Soak 1 cup hulled sesame seeds overnight. Drain, rinse, and put them in a blender with 2 cups (400 ml) pure water. Blend for 90 seconds and strain through a fine-wire mesh strainer. To the strained sesame milk, add 1 frozen banana, 1 package of frozen blueberries 12 ounces, 1 tablespoon (15 ml) agave nectar, and $1/4$ teaspoon (1 ml) vanilla. Blend 90 seconds and serve. Enjoy.

Optional: You may freeze this mixture in ice cube trays with popsicle sticks as blueberry creamy pops for a spring and summer treat.

Lunch Sunday

ALFALFA SPROUTS SALAD OR NORI ROLLS

Ingredients

1 cup (200 ml) alfalfa sprouts

1 cup (200 ml) lettuce of your choice, chopped

½ cup (100 ml) each chopped celery, avocado, and tomatoes

Spices of your choice, plus 1 tablespoon (15 ml) of Bragg Aminos, if you'd like.

Directions

Mix all ingredients and eat as salad or roll in nori sheets.

Dinner Sunday

TUNA (NOT) SALAD STACKERS

Ingredients

1 tablespoon (15 ml) dulse, kelp, or any other sea vegetable, finely chopped

2 cucumbers, thinly sliced

2 cups (400 ml) salad greens

Optional: Collard greens, tomato, red bell pepper, celery stalks.

Directions

Use paté from Wednesday and add to each cup of left over dulse, kelp, or another sea vegetable. Slather cucumber slices with any pate recipe made from soaked, blended sunflower seeds, garlic, and herbs. You may also make a wrap with collard greens to which you add sliced avocado, or stuff a tomato, red bell pepper, or celery stalks. Serve with salad greens with dressing of your choice.

Note about beverage selections: Some people feel it is best if beverages are consumed at least half an hour before or after a meal. Serve these dishes with purified water or your choice of herbal teas, including alfalfa, Pau D'Arco, chamomile, ginger, and yerba mate. Bitters teas are best consumed just prior to meals.

SALAD DRESSINGS

PAPAYA SEED DRESSING

Yield: Makes $1^1/_2$ cups (300 ml)

$1^1/_2$ tablespoons (23 ml) fresh papaya seeds

1 cup (200 ml) olive oil

$^1/_3$ cup (68 ml) lemon juice or apple cider vinegar

1 tablespoon (15 ml) fresh lime juice

2 teaspoons (10 ml) agave nectar and 2 teaspoons (10 ml) minced onion

$^1/_2$ teaspoon (3 ml) sea salt

$^1/_2$ teaspoon (3 ml) dry mustard

Directions

Place all ingredients except papaya seeds in a blender. Blend 2 minutes at high speed. Add papaya seeds and blend until mixture is thick and the seeds look like ground pepper. Chill.

Notes: Some people save and dry their papaya seeds and grind them fine to use as pepper or additional spice for foods. Papaya seeds are also known to act as a vermifuge to kill certain gastrointestinal parasites; pumpkin seeds have a similar effect. They are known to scratch the skin of tapeworms so that other vermifuges may enter the skin of the parasite; the pumpkin also acts as a mild hypnotic that causes the tape worm's grip to release.

SIMPLE SALAD DRESSING

Ingredients

1 cup (200 ml) extra-virgin olive oil

$^1/_4$ cup (50 ml) flax or toasted sesame oil

1 raw garlic clove

$^1/_4$ cup (50 ml) fresh-squeezed lemon or lime juice

2 tablespoons (30 ml) fresh chopped herbs of your choice or 1 tablespoon (15 ml) Italian herbs

4 tablespoons (60 ml) either Bragg Aminos, wheat-free tamari, or Nama Shoyu

Directions

Mix all ingredients in a glass jar and shake well.

SELENIUM HOT DOGS

Ingredients

1 large organic raw date, pit removed

1 Brazil nut (high in selenium)

Directions

Stuff the date with the Brazil nut. Eat and enjoy as a high-energy snack. Only 1 daily.

RAW CACAO COOKIES

Ingredients

2 cups (400 ml) walnuts

1 cup (200 ml) pecans or almonds or sunflower seeds, soaked 4 hours

8–10 dates or 1$\frac{1}{2}$ cups (300 ml), soaked 1–4 hours

$\frac{1}{2}$ cup (100 ml) cacao nibs

Variation: Add 2 teaspoons (10 ml) vanilla or almond extract, a pinch of sea salt, $\frac{1}{2}$ cup (100 ml) grated coconut, 1 tablespoon (15 ml) cinnamon, $\frac{1}{4}$ teaspoon (1 ml) nutmeg. Half a cup (100 ml) of raisins or $\frac{1}{4}$ cup (50 ml) agave nectar may be added, if you want a sweeter cookie.

Directions

Blend all ingredients in a food processor with an S-blade just until crumbly. Stir in cacao nibs. Take a tablespoon and roll the mixture into a small ball. You may flatten this to make this more cookie-like. Refrigerate. It keeps well for a long time. Do not eat more than two at a time because they may cause blood sugar or pH issues.

Final Words of Support

To exist is to change; to change is to mature;
to mature is to create oneself endlessly.

—HENRI BERGSON

Make this healing lifestyle an adventure. Have fun with this new information about what food is and does. It's just the beginning of your new
quality of life. You will learn other perspectives and attitudes, even within the
raw foods community. Notice how well your body responds to this new way
of nurturing yourself. Love yourself enough to heal. Every food choice should
be a conscious, considerate choice.

There are critics of the raw food diet. Some of these critics may even be in
your own family or among your friends. People are eager to protect the status
quo or support the misinformation created by a profit-oriented junk food
industry. Some people may not appreciate the fact that you are losing weight
on your raw diet or getting healthier. The best way to judge this diet is to try it
for three months and see how you feel. Document the changes that you notice
inside and out. There are raw food restaurants as well as raw food groups so
you can interact socially with others who are benefiting from this new healing
lifestyle. I would caution you to avoid joining a raw foods cult or following
any raw foods guru to obsession. Study and learn what you can from others.
Give raw foods a chance, and stick with the raw eating regimen. Cravings are
natural, since acidic food is one on the most addictive substances on earth. Eat
more greens if you feel hungry.

If you find the information that I have shared useful, please pass it on.

Share this book and check my website for a list of my upcoming speaking and teaching engagements. I'd love to meet you and hear your healing story. It has been my privilege to share this information with you. Remember: every healthy choice you make every day about each bite you take will allow you to enjoy a vibrant life.

I have frequently been asked at presentations and classes if a raw foods diet can be dangerous. In my forty-some years of nutritional studies and personal experience, I have gained the clear understanding that one of the most dangerous diets on the planet is one that is high in processed foods, hormone- and antibiotic-laden dairy products, and animal protein, and low in raw vegetables and plant-based foods. You do not have to look far to find someone who is suffering the ill effects of what is called the Standard American Diet. Obesity is an epidemic in America. We are left at a cultural disadvantage because most of the educational materials about diet are rife with confusing, conflicting information that comes from special interest groups. By taking the responsibility to study good nutrition and paying attention to how our bodies respond to certain foods, we can create a healthier future not only for ourselves but for generations to come. I challenge you to try my 4-3-2-1 raw healing diet for three months, and discover how rewarding and simple it can be. Live each day of your life in your own Blue Zone. You can eat better foods because you do matter and your life is important.

Be well and happy,
Dr. Karyn Mitchell

References

Adams, Mike. "Natural Diet Lowers Disease Risk after Just 30 Days, Study Finds." (December 12, 2010). Naturalnews.com.

Airola, Paavo. *How to Keep Slim, Healthy and Young With Juice Fasting* Sherwood, OR: Health Plus Publishers, 1971.

Bergner, Paul. *The Healing Power of Minerals.* Roseville, CA: Prima Lifestyles Publishing, 1997.

Boutenko, Victoria. *12 Steps to End Your Addiction to Cooked Food.* Berkeley, CA: North Atlantic Books, 2007.

————. *Green for Life.* Ashland, OR: Raw Family Publishing, 2005.

Brotman, Juliano & Erika Lenkert. *Raw: The Uncook Book: New Vegetarian Food for Life.* New York: Regan Books, 1999.

Brownstein, Dr. David. *Iodine: Why You Need It, Why You Can't Live Without It.* West Bloomfield, MI: Medical Alternatives Press, 2004

Buettner, Dan. *The Blue Zones: Lessons for Living Longer from People Who've Lived the Longest.* Washington, DC: National Geographic, 2008.

Cousens, Dr. Gabriel, M.D. *Conscious Eating.* Berkeley, CA: North Atlantic Books, 2005.

————. *There Is a Cure for Diabetes: The Tree of Life 21-Day+ Program.* Berkeley, CA: North Atlantic Books, 2008.

Damrau, Frederic, M.D. *The Medical Annals of the District of Columbia.* Washington, DC: Medical Society of the District of Columbia, 1961.

Elliott, Angela. *Alive in 5: Raw Gourmet Meals in Five Minutes.* Summertown, TN: Book Publishing Company, 2007.

Erasmus, Udo. *Fats That Heal, Fats That Kill: The Complete Guide to Fats, Oils, Cholesterol and Human Health.* Burnaby, BC, Canada: Alive Books 1993.

Etkin, Nina. *Edible Medicines.* Tucson: University of Arizona Press, 2006.

Fife, Bruce, ND. *The Healing Miracles of Coconut Oil.* New York: Penguin Group, 1999.

Ford, Debbie. *The Dark Side of the Light Chasers.* New York: Berkley Publishing Co., 1998.

Fuhrman, Joel, M.D. *Eat to Live.* New York: Little, Brown and Co., 2003.

Galbraith, John Kenneth. *The Affluent Society.* New York: Houghton Mifflin Co., 1958.

Gershon, Michael, M.D. *The Second Brain.* New York: HarperCollins, 1998.

Hawaii Farm Bureau Federation. *Hawaii Farmers Market Cookbook: Fresh Island Products from A to Z.* Honolulu: Watermark Publishing, 2006.

Howell, Dr. Edward, M.D. *The Status of Food Enzymes in Digestion and Metabolism.* Twin Lakes, WI: Lotus Press, 1946.

———. *Enzyme Nutrition.* New York: Penguin Putman, Inc., 1985.

Jensen, Bernard, DC. *650 Prize Winning Blender Recipes for Nutrition-Minded People: Blending Magic.* Escondido, CA: Bernard Jensen, 1958.

———. *Chlorella: Gem of the Orient.* Escondido, CA: Bernard Jensen, 1987.

Johns, Timothy, Ph.D. *The Origins of Human Diet and Medicine.* Tucson: The University of Arizona Press, 1996.

Kushi, Michio & Alex Jack. *The Macrobiotic Path to Total Health: A Complete Guide to Naturally Preventing and Relieving More Than 200 Chronic Conditions and Disorders.* New York: Ballantine, 2004.

Lee, William H., and Michael Rosenbaum. *Chlorella.* New York: McGraw-Hill, 1987.

McDougall, John A., M.D. *The McDougall Program.* New York: Penguin Group, 1990.

Mindell, Earl. *The Vitamin Bible.* New York: Time Warner Book Group, 2004.

Mehl-Madrona, Lewis, M.D. *Coyote Medicine.* New York: Fireside, 1998.

Nearing, Helen & Scott. *The Good Life: Helen and Scott Nearing's Sixty Years of Self-Sufficient Living.* New York: Schocken Books, 1990.

Null, Gary, Ph.D. *The Vegetarian Handbook: Eating Right for Total Health.* New York: St. Martin's/Griffin, 1996.

Patenaude, Frederic. *Sunfood Cuisine: A Practical Guide to Raw Vegetarian Cuisine.* San Diego: Nature's First Law, 2003.

Phillip, John. "Diet Makes All the Difference with Pancreatic Cancer Risk" (November 18, 2010). Naturalnews.com.

Pitchford, Paul. *Healing with Whole Foods: Asian Traditions and Modern Nutrition.* Berkeley, CA: North Atlantic Books, 2003.

Pollan, Michael. *The Omnivore's Dilemma.* New York: Penguin Press, 2006.

Rhio. *Hooked on Raw.* New York: Beso Entertainment, 2000.

Rudell, Wendy. *The Raw Transformation: Energizing Your Life with Living Foods.* Berkeley, CA: North Atlantic Books, 2006.

Robbins, John. *May All Be Fed.* New York: Morrow, 1992.

Roe, Daphne, M.D. *Drug Induced Nutritional Deficiencies.* Westport, CT: AVI Publishing, 1976.

Safron, Jeremy. *The Raw Truth: The Art of Preparing Living Foods.* Berkeley, CA: Celestial Arts, 2003.

Sellmeyer, Dr. Deborah. "Osteoporosis, Conditions and Treatments." UCSF Medical Center (October 9, 2010). www.uscfhealth.org.

Shannon, Nomi. *The Raw Gourmet.* Burnaby, BC, Canada: Alive Books, 1999.

Servan-Schreiber, Dr. David. "David Servan-Schriber on Cheating Death." *Psychology Today* (April 2009): 108.

Shelton, Herbert & Ronald G. Cridland. *Fasting Can Save Your Life.* San Antonio: American Natural Hygiene Society, 1978.

———. *Fasting for Renewal of Life.* Tampa, FL: National Health Association, 1974.

Turner, Victor. *Liminality, Kabbalah, and the Media.* Burlington, MA: Academic Press, 1985.

"USDA Table of Nutrient Retention Factors 2003." www.USDA.gov/wps/portal/.

Watts, Dr. Meriel. *Pesticides and Breast Cancer: A Wake Up Call.* www.cancer.org/cancer/breastcancer/detailedguide/breast-cancer-risk-factors.

Wigmore, Ann. *Recipes for Longer Life.* Wayne, NJ: Avery Publishing Group, Inc., 1978.

———. *Why Suffer: How I Overcame Illness and Pain Naturally.* New York: Avery, 1985.

Willett, Walter, M.D., & P. J. Skerrett. *Eat, Drink, and Be Healthy: The Harvard Medical School Guide to Healthy Eating.* New York: Free Press, 2005.

Resources

American Journal of Clinical Nutrition
www.ajcn.org/

Environmental Working Group
www.ewg.org/pesticidesorganics

Genova Diagnostics Laboratory
www.genovadiagnostics.com

Journal of the American Medical Association
www.Jama.ama-assn.org/ cgi/content/abstract/287/23/3127

Mayo Clinic
www.MayoClinic.com/health/supplements/NU00198

Not Milk
www.notmilk.com

Nutrition Review
www.nutritionreview.org/

U.S. Centers for Disease Control
www.cdc.gov/nchs/

Index

About the Author

Dr. **Karyn Mitchell** is a naturopathic doctor with a Ph.D. in psychology. She has attended the University of Iowa, the University of Nebraska, Loras College, Buena Vista College, Midwest College of Naturopathic Medicine, and Westbrook University. After receiving her doctorate in psychology, she pursued a degree in naturopathy. She attended a year of training and certification with Foundations in Herbal Medicine with Tierrona LowDog, M.D. After she received her naturopathic degree from Midwest College, she continued her education in herbal pharmacology by taking courses at Bastyr University. She was involved in research concerning women's health and cancer for Midwest College of Naturopathic Medicine. Advanced studies in parasitology and AIDS led her twice to Mexico for a research project concerning the work of Dr. Hulda Clark. Dr. Mitchell has continued her education by completing coursework offered by the American Botanical Council. She studied homeopathy at the Devon School in England. She is board-certified as a traditional naturopath. She is involved in autoimmune and raw diet research and education.

A former high school English teacher, Dr. Mitchell earned a BA in English at the University of Iowa. She has won postgraduate awards for writing in fiction and poetry.

She is an international teacher and speaker in the fields of nutrition; iridology; natural medicine; Reiki; hypnotherapy; the vegetarian, vegan, and raw foods lifestyle; and shamanism. She has been a keynote speaker at many national events, including Whole Life Expos and the Raw Spirit Festival in Sedona, Arizona. She has been a student of psychology, natural health, and philosophy for over thirty-eight years.

Dr. Mitchell has devoted her life's work to helping others address their healing process. She maintains an office at Haven Holistic Center in St. Charles, Illinois, and works as a naturopath and therapist. She has taught at two high schools and three universities in the United States. She is currently acting president and a professor at Midwest College of Naturopathic Medicine, teaching advanced laboratory courses in anatomy, herbology, homeopathy, nutrition, women's health, laboratory testing, iridology, and deep tissue lymphatic drainage.

Dr. Mitchell has written four books concerning natural healing and one work of fiction. She also has three audio CDs, titled *Heal Now, Raw 4-3-2-1 Healing Diet,* and *Reboot Your Brain.* She is most proud of her family as well as the dedicated students who have studied with her.

As a teacher in natural health, Dr. Mitchell is comforted to know that the future of traditional medicine and healing belongs to those who care compassionately for others and are diligent enough to learn the basic truth about healthy living. Many diseases begin with food intolerances that are neither recognized nor diagnosed. Food can be our medicine, and medicine can be our food. Eat lots of raw, fresh fruits and vegetables to get healing enzymes, and eat only organic whenever possible.

Karyn Mitchell, ND, Ph.D.
email: mitchell1972@comcast.net
Website: www.drmitchellnd.com
603 Geneva Road
St. Charles, IL 60174
Phone: 815-732-7150
Fax: 630-443-9930